"The paramount purpose of this book
is to point you toward joy."

•

The joy of being alive and beautiful . . .
Yours from The Golden Door.

•

"When I get my stomach flattened
and my head straightened, things just
seem to come together nicely."
—Barbara Howar

•

"I do it three times a year
to save my life."
—Bill Blass

•

"I felt better than I ever had
in my whole life."
—Fashion Model Cristina Delorean

•

"Will increase your happiness
and personal growth."
—Kim Novak

•

"It was incredible!
I had a sense of being healthy.
I felt happy."
—Calvin Klein

Revised Edition

SECRETS
OF THE
GOLDEN DOOR

by Deborah Szekely Mazzanti

Dedicated to Edmond Bordeaux Szekely, teacher, philosopher, and impossible man, whom I met in 1933, married in 1939, and divorced in 1969; who gave me my life's work and my two children.

Dedicated also to the 250,000 people who have crossed my threshold and who have taught me even as I taught them. Their trust inspired me to seek the answers reprinted within these pages.

And with a Special Word for both my children, Alex and Livia Szekely, and Vincent E. Mazzanti, my husband. Their love sustains me and their pride in me makes me do my very best.

SECRETS OF THE GOLDEN DOOR

A Bantam Book

PRINTING HISTORY

William Morrow edition published July 1977
2nd printing . . . August 1977
3rd printing . . . August 1977

Literary Guild selection January 1978

Serialized in Family Health December 1977

Serialized in Cosmopolitan April 1978

Serialized in Redbook January 1978

Serialized in Woman's Digest March 1978

Revised Bantam edition / September 1979

ISBN 0-553-12695-4

Published simultaneously in the United States and Canada

Bantam Books are published by Bantam Books, Inc. Its trademark, consisting of the words "Bantam Books" and the portrayal of a bantam, is Registered in U.S. Patent and Trademark Office and in other countries. Marca Registrada. Bantam Books, Inc., 666 Fifth Avenue, New York, New York 10019

PRINTED IN THE UNITED STATES OF AMERICA

0 9 8 7 6 5 4 3 2

*Happiness is difficult to find within,
impossible to find elsewhere.*

—SEBASTIEN CHAMFORT

(Copied from the flyleaf of *The Dictionary
of Love,* given to me on my fourteenth birthday
by Edmond Bordeaux Szekely.)

ACKNOWLEDGMENTS

With grateful thanks to Ned Riley, Livia Szekely, and John Poppy, who tidied my reams of untidy notes, and to Roberta Ridgely, who made it all so readable.

To Charles Schneider, who has been the Golden Door photographer since before we opened.

To Chris Silkwood, exercise director of the Golden Door; and to Kathryn Scott of her department, who posed for the photographs in the exercise section.

To Michel Stroot, Rae Piper, and Jinx Morgan for their contribution to the menus and recipes in Chapter IX.

To Robert Mosher, AIA, who designed the Golden Door with all the subtlety of his art, making it an integral factor in the joy, the quiet discipline, and the unobtrusive beauty—in short, the "otherness"— which Golden Door guests come seeking.

CONTENTS

PREFACE TO
THE BANTAM EDITION

Today as I conclude the revision of my book, we live in a changed world. The unchallenged bestseller—deservedly, I think—is *The Complete Book of Running*. And the gladdest tiding in your daily newspaper enumerates the growing numbers who exercise daily, or otherwise reflects our rising national concern for real food, real vitality, and for coming to real (not half-hearted) terms with existence.

All this amounts to the most overwhelming U.S. phenomenon which has taken place within your lifetime or mine. I can think of no comparable movement sweeping this country without benefit of a multimillion-dollar budget for promotion and advertising.

When Bantam Books gave me carte blanche to revise my book for the paperback edition, I fortunately already had the advantage of reader reaction (how can I ever give enough thanks to those people who took the time to write me!) plus the gratification of seeing what *U.S. News & World Report* in early 1974 had dismissed as a "fitness kick" and by early 1978 was terming a "fitness mania." (Some others have employed the expression "fitness epidemic." This seems to me particularly inapt. Our new interest in maintaining healthy bodies is more to be equated with a spontaneous; drugless, painless, epidemic-forestalling, nationwide vaccination campaign.)

Since the 5,000,000 joggers of two years ago have swelled their kinetic ranks to at least 25,000,000, some of whom got their start at the Golden Door or Rancho La Puerta, one new chapter is devoted to jogging—one might say by popular demand.

This book has been reworked page by page; the longer I live, the more I learn about the interaction of mind, body, exercise, and nutrition. With the exception of the office-chair exercises, all the exercises in this edition are new, and that section has been greatly amplified. Now it gives much attention to the daily stretches that preserve and/or restore flexibility. I see flexibility and youth as synonymous, whether for the body or the mind-body. Adopting such attitudes, I feel, is what equips us for "living for life."

"How to be Healthy, Happy, Self-ful" is another new chapter which offers guidance for the woman who now has to make her way in what has been called (I wish it hadn't been) the Me Generation.

As for the final one-third of the book, comprising the recipes and menus, it carries just a few minor changes. This section remains intact not only because of the many people who continue to tell me, "I keep just two cookbooks in my kitchen—yours and one other," but because of a worldwide poll recently conducted by Dr. Kaare R. Norum of the Institute for Nutrition Research, University of Oslo School of Medicine. Results prove that, despite an occasional sensational news story to the contrary, no basic disagreement exists among the world's leading nutrition researchers. Of 193 respondents, 188 stated their conviction that diet affects the heart. And 92% expressed the opinion that a diet change is indicated for affluent societies throughout the world.

This confirms the empirical knowledge I've accumulated in years of challenging people to adopt a new and better life-style. (The total of the guests I've worked with must be approaching half a million. Hard for you to conceive? Hard for me to believe, too!) I'm no longer a lonely voice crying out in the wilderness. And I can give you positive assurance that this health philosophy which I've spent a lifetime preparing in order to pass on to you, represents no fad of the moment. Think of it as a trusted friend you can turn to this year, and the next, and the next, as you learn to eat and move and live for life.

A NOTE
FROM THE AUTHOR

The best way to begin our time together is for me to tell you something about myself, because the Golden Door is such an intensely personal extension of me—of what I have learned in fifty-six years of growing up in the health field (in what today is called holistic health). This projection of my life's experiences into the Golden Door is what has made it unique among spas. Since 1940, my life's work has been to see that my guests carry home the conviction and the know-how to live and to grow with more life, for more years.

I suppose the first chapter of my adult life began in 1940, when my husband, Professor Edmond Bordeaux Szekely, and I (a bride just one month past eighteen) drove down a dusty corrugated road leading to an old Spanish land grant in Baja California, Mexico, called

Rancho La Puerta ("Ranch of the Door"). We sat on silver plush upholstery in an only slightly dilapidated 1928 Cadillac with cut-crystal bud vases between its side windows; it towed a handmade, silver-plated trailer box which contained all our worldly goods.

There, at Rancho La Puerta, we pioneered the basic approach to exercising and eating that would later become famous. We did this by developing the Activity Day. Till then few had considered how to replace the missing ingredient in modern life that once was the prerequisite for all living beings—continuous movement. To gather food, primitive man and animal alike were preoccupied with a dawn-to-dusk search. We translated this dawn-to-dusk migration into the Activity Day. And this is fundamental to the fantastic results that have made the Golden Door world-famous.

It is a weird feeling to be required to explain how you came upon an original approach. At one point many years ago I began by saying to myself, "Here we are in the age of enlightenment. Why then the lack of well-being? Is it that we are leading our lives as if our bodies didn't really exist? What would be the most sensible means of readjustment?"

That I should have asked such questions and looked for answers was not surprising in view of my experience. I had neither medical training nor degree. But I possessed a one-of-a-kind background in exploring theories of health and natural living.

I must have been four years old when my mother became a vice-president of the New York Vegetarian Society. That would make the year 1926. Besides being vegetarian, my family also was fruitarian—meaning we ate nothing but raw fruits, vegetables, and nuts.

Almost every weekend we hiked to a different health camp. Midweek I fell asleep listening to health lectures all over Manhattan.

When I was seven, in 1929, the impact of the Great Depression hit us—but differently than it hit most New Yorkers. There wasn't much for fruitarians to eat. Of course, we too were suddenly poor, and many fresh fruits and nuts became not only expensive, but simply unavailable. Faced with a choice between starvation or relinquishing their principles, my parents decided to spend what money was left on steamship tickets. We sailed to Tahiti.

When my parents placed me in a convent school before going off to assess the other islands, they didn't realize that no one there spoke English. The school's everyday language was Tahitian; its second official language was French. Somehow I got through my first day at the convent without mishap. I credit my successes since that time to my exceptional vitality and my ability to observe. I guess it all began at that school in Tahiti, because there I had to learn not by listening, but by watching.

It was while we were in Tahiti that we met Professor Edmond Bordeaux Szekely. He had spent his youth researching early civilizations and searching for ways to apply natural living to an increasingly unnatural culture. He became the strongest influence in the life of my family. When we left the South Pacific after four and a half years, we were determined to live only half of each year in a city, and to spend the other half in a primitive community.

We spent many summers in Professor Szekely's health camps. This took us from Lake Elsinore in southern California to Rio Corona in Tamaulipas, Mexico. I spent my teen-age years listening to the small but motley group (health tramps and peers of the realm, faddists and scholars) who then comprised the health enthusiasts of the world.

I graduated from high school in 1938, when I was just sixteen. My mother decided that I was too young for college. Instead, I followed my family to Central Mexico, where Professor Szekely had now set up a new health camp. Joining him, we learned that his secretary had just been called home to England by the death of his father. Since the Professor was totally helpless about day-to-day practical details, I pitched in to help and remained after my parents returned to California. I proved such an efficient secretary and aide that, when my parents wrote to say it was time for me to return home to resume my education, he married me. That was 1939; we were to remain married until 1969.

Back to 1940: Professor Szekely was concerned both about the impending expiration of his U.S. immigration visa and by whispered rumors concerning probable internment of aliens if America should be drawn into the Second World War. A captain in the Romanian reserves who was now a man without a country, he chose to emigrate to Mexico. A happy and obedient new wife, I accompanied him. Together, on June 6, 1940, we opened our first spa, Rancho La Puerta, in Tecate, Baja California. As I have said, this was when my adult life really began.

From the beginning we experimented. We read and discussed and tried every health discipline and diet theory you're hearing about now: bean sprouts and acidophilus milk, total fasting and interval fasting, the grape cure, the mucus-free diet, morning walks, and mud baths. I have never come across anything that we didn't try once. Today every so-called new diet plan or exercise idea is, to me, *déjà vu.* Direct observation is the key to everything I've learned.

Rancho La Puerta, the Golden Door's forerunner, grew and grew, eventually expanding into the largest health resort of its kind. By now, almost a quarter of a million guests have stepped through its welcoming archway.

I celebrated our twentieth wedding anniversary by opening the Golden Door, a resort planned from the start to be small, intimate, and my version of heaven. We began with only twelve guests each week. (Even today we remain the world's smallest major spa.) But after a time our marriage began to falter, and in 1969 we were divorced.

Another milestone, my fiftieth birthday, marked the beginning of Book II in my life. On that date—May 3, 1972—I became engaged to Vincent E. Mazzanti, the wise and warm and wonderfully understanding psychoanalyst whom I married in June. And in that same year I reached the decision to build a new Golden Door; over thirty years of experience and dreams were poured into an establishment which was to be hailed as "the ultimate spa."

Today the Golden Door accepts just thirty guests at any one time, so that our staff of eighty-seven can give the most meticulous attention to each one. The location, in a beautiful little southern California valley, affords both seclusion and almost year-round sunshine. In such ideally protective surroundings one can dare to advance new ideas and concepts.

All our guests take out into the world heightened vitality—the desire and ability to create a new self, to live more and more in a world of his or her own choosing.

My dearest hope is that this is what will happen to you as you read this book.

DEBORAH SZEKELY MAZZANTI

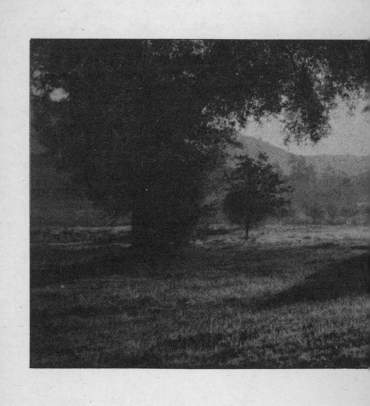

CHAPTER I

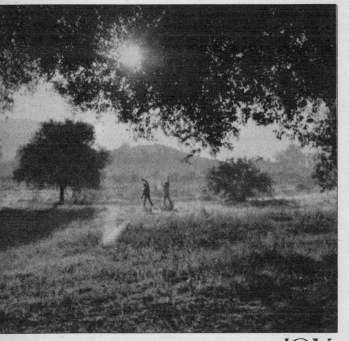

JOY,
THE SECRET
INGREDIENT

The paramount purpose of this book is to point you toward joy—whether by talking about getting to know your body, feeling it as one with Nature, or about cooking some of the most delicious food you've ever tasted. Joy is what our guests come seeking at the Golden Door, and it is what they take home. It's the secret I want you to make your own as you read these pages.

What I'm about to tell you is as much a matter of context for your life and its varying aspects as it is a matter of content. Absorb everything in your own time, in your own way, and in your own sequence. A valid program must accommodate itself to the swirling patterns of my guests' everyday lives after they are home again—and to your daily activities.

HEALTH-TO-GO

Years go by, names change, but people and their problems remain the same. The Golden Door program has been shared by such widely divergent personalities as Sally Quinn and Barbra Streisand; Roberta Flack and Cher; Bess Myerson and Dyan Cannon; Shana Alexander and Natalie Wood; Barbara Howar and Phyllis George; the Gabors—mother Jolie and daughters Eva and Zsa Zsa; and the forever young and forever active such as Debbie Reynolds and Dinah Shore. During Men's Weeks, our notables have ranged from Robert Wagner and Cliff Robertson to George Kennedy and William Holden; Bill Blass and Stanley Kramer and Paul Anka to the late Aldous Huxley.

Those who return again and again, and seem to grow increasingly luminous with each visit, are the ones who have married their lives to a healthful year-round schedule based on Golden Door guidelines.

IT'S A BALANCING ACT

There's nothing really mysterious about these secrets that will stimulate you and give you so much verve. But you and the program you adopt for yourself must be characterized by balance rather than by overzealousness.

Trust me. At one extreme are depression, boredom, and fatigue; the Cookie Monster; obesity; and, eventually, alarming symptoms. At the opposite pole are Captain Bligh, nose to the grindstone, shoulder to the wheel, and *Achtung!* Aren't you relieved you'll be asked only to effect an appropriate balance between them? *Le juste milieu* is what the French call it, the point between two extremes—another name for the Golden Mean, another name for keeping things in perspective, and another name for the Golden Door.

As the Golden Door philosophy is revealed to you, you'll recognize the profound relationship of your body, mind, and spirit. For many, this new relationship may be like a trip to a foreign land. When you begin such a trip you bring along a simple vocabulary, maps, and guidebooks. And these are what I intend to supply you with in this book—my secrets of the Golden Door.

YOUR PERSONAL
FINE-TUNER

First off, I am going to help you to learn to listen and look, intently and intensively. Begin with your own reflection in the mirror. Would you say it shows someone who is strong, kinetic, functioning smoothly with all systems Go? Then you can be sure the same is true of what is going on inside your psyche and mind-body.

But if your reflection is otherwise, that too is an incisive report on your inner state.

Observe, interpret, listen to voices from within, whether you are communicating with partner, friends, children, or your own mind/body self.

With this in mind, while you are still in bed and not really quite awake, here is what you must do just before you rise each morning, exactly as we do at the Golden Door. Take a moment to feel your body, all of it. This was and is your "In the beginning . . ." (Alas, more darkly, it also can be your "Finis.") Count your fingers and toes just as you would a newborn baby's. (All there?)

CHECK YOUR BODY
THOROUGHLY BECAUSE
YOU CAN'T CHECK OUT OF IT

This is your home, where your mind/body live. Your body is your permanent home, not a motel. You can't check out of it and leave it on the bed this morning. You can't move out forever when you are forty or fifty because it doesn't suit you anymore.

You are aware that each day of your life is a blank page, stretching out before you, waiting for you to fill it in. Think of your body's kinetic energy as the pen that authors your history. Your pen can be full of bold strokes and handsome paragraph beginnings. It can move along steadily with a controlled, vital flow. Or it can splutter, blot, fail, and be tossed aside.

Now you are ready to make note of the date at the top that identifies this day's page—first, with two minutes of stretching and moving exercises, nude. Exercise before a full-length mirror, with your eyes wide open. Start at the top; slowly stretch, first push out the world with your hands and arms, and then embrace the world, tightly, enfolding your arms. Feel your freedom, breathe deeply, be aware of the air touching you, wiggle your toes, and identify the movement of each one. This feeling of wholeness, this sense of the mind/body in which you live with your inner and outer self, is what you are going to use to create your day and your entire life.

Hop quickly on the scales, for in planning your day you need to know whether yesterday built up your fuel reserves or depleted them.

YOUR CLASSY ACTION SUIT

Do not put on your robe, I implore you. It speaks of relaxation, great for the evening hours, the end of the day in which you have worked long and hard. It insidiously suggests that you are tired, so why not sit down and take it easy. It says everything can wait while poor you has a second cup of coffee. Of course you are tired, you just spent six or seven or eight hours in bed. Now is the time for the swing of the pendulum, the time for movement after non-movement; consider the surge of the ocean after the ebb of the tide.

So on with your jogging suit, for it carries implicit messages of high stepping and high gear. It is your commitment to yourself. Keep it on while you square away the beds and the breakfast dishes in jig time. Or jog time.

If you are one of the lucky ones who can exercise before breakfast, that's ideal. If you're a houseperson, you may have to wait till the kids are off to school and everyone has left. If you work, you will have to set your alarm thirty minutes earlier. Believe me when I say a half-hour spent in exercise does far more for you than that last half-hour passed in sleep.

SAME TIME, NEXT YEAR

It's your exercise routine that will get your day off to its real start. The important thing about exercise is that it becomes a daily habit, as much a reflex as breathing. You establish that by picking a time slot, a permanent one about which you never have to make any day-to-day decisions. After all, you weren't born with a toothbrush at your fingertips; yet you brush your teeth at least twice a day without thinking. The kind of exercise you choose and the length of the exercise period are dealt with later in this book. Now I'm merely talking about the concept—the creation of a reflex, your own reeducation.

Schedule your morning exercise program for Monday through Friday. Your Saturday and Sunday schedule can be fitted into your weekend plans. Exercise in the morning has many physiological and psychological benefits. Perhaps it has something to do with the rising of the sun, the singing of the birds, the lifting of the mist, and even the tug of the tides. There's a great uplift in the morning, gathering one's strengths, marshaling one's energies—all combining to help you enter your day with a strong feeling that you surround the day's tasks rather than the other way around.

For me the greatest benefit of morning exercise is the return home from the park, the feeling that God's in His heaven and all's right with the world. You will feel energized because you have set a goal and then achieved it with ease. This confidence will carry over into everything you do. I believe it's no coincidence that my friends who walk and jog and exercise invariably are the people of greatest achievement.

YOU CAN REVIVE
TWILIGHT SAVING TIME

Just as you use exercise to get yourself up in the morning, also use it to wind down at night. There once was a time called twilight, the prelude for what many people feel is the most rewarding time of day—the evening. The work required for daily life was then completed, and people could live a little for themselves; we must recreate that bridge between the day's activities and the night's different pace.

When you arrive home, instead of switching on television and pouring a drink, put on your jogging shoes, run around the block for ten minutes. Or swim. Or hop onto your stationary bicycle, conveniently parked in front of the TV set for all to use. Or just step into the back bedroom for ten minutes of alternating exercise and jump-rope. It's not important exactly what you do; the important thing is to vary the pattern of tension and the pattern of breathing. But I will get to all this later. For now, remember your three daily exercise periods, one at the beginning of your day, then a couple of licks and a promise—an energy break at noon—followed by a little wind-down burst at day's end.

AT BREAKFAST, PLOT YOUR COURSES FOR LUNCH AND DINNER

Back to your breakfast. At the table plan your day—not only its activities but the fuel necessary to power those activities. Look at your breakfast plate and think of the food before you as so much quality energy. This serving represents tennis, this the exercise you did this morning, and this the hours you'll be seated at your desk.

Compose your daily shopping list at breakfast. Project an accurate calendar for your whole day. Mark your lunch plans—whether you're having lunch out or just a cup of yogurt at your desk—and at the same time think about dinner. If you're a twosome, both of you should consider not only this evening's dinner but what your social schedule for the week will be. A big meal on Wednesday means a small meal on Thursday. Plan your meals with the same perspective as you do your other activities.

Breakfast in itself is simple. You'll find out all about that in the nutrition chapter and in the recipes that follow (pages 241–385).

WIN AT LUNCH
WITH A TRIPLE PLAY

For lunch, have three courses—an appetite-spoiler, an exercise break, and lunch. Your appetite-spoiler should be eaten thirty minutes before your meal, either at home or at your desk before you walk briskly to the restaurant. Its purpose is to lift your blood sugar (again, I'll amplify later). Then, for the restaurant eater, if you wish to lose weight, choose your lunch from the appetizers, the hors d'oeuvres; you will find these portions are quite small. At home eat a health-and-life-giving low-calorie lunch; visualize the quality of the energy in every food. You will soon find you do not cherish the image of looking and feeling like a doughnut.

DINNER—ONE SIZE
DOES NOT FIT ALL

Dinner is the principal meal—the main event. There are many tricks to making the ritual of dinner psychologically and physiologically satisfying; you will learn about them later. But beware of the notion of portion control. Most cookbooks and restaurants deal in calories sufficient to feed a rather large and active man. Cruise-ship menus provide enough calories to power a man six feet, eight inches tall who weighs two hundred sixty pounds. If you went on such a cruise ship and stayed long enough, you would never measure that man's height, but you certainly could approach his weight.

I'm going to help you find the way to put the right amount of food on your plate in the first place, so that, after your meal, you will not feel that you've denied yourself anything. I cannot give you X-ray vision so that when you look at a dish you see the total calories. But I will tell you how you can come close to this. And I will provide you with a workable, companionable sort of guide so that you'll know when it's a day to be very, very good; or when the day's been rough and it's o.k. to eat a little more and soothe your ruffled feathers.

FACE IT, FOOD IS PERPETUAL EMOTION

From infancy on people have developed the habit of cry, food, cry, food. The baby cries. The mother soothes and feeds. Today, whenever you're unhappy, it makes perfect sense that you should want to eat, to unwind, to relax, to be stroked. This is not a habit you are going to lose, but you'll learn how to make capital of it by assuring that everything you do eat gives you maximum psychological and physiological pleasure. Only then will you find genuine satisfaction without guilt —and with a new awareness.

STRIP YOUR SHOPPING CART FOR ACTION

This awareness will lead you to selecting and choos-ing quality food because a life of high vitality needs a high-octane fuel. Our Saturday-go-to-the-supermarket shopping style is a direct descendant of those Satur-days when people hitched up the buckboard and went into town to do the marketing, to trade the surplus eggs for flour, and to buy the oil and the sugar and the few other basics not grown at home. But in those days food was fresh and unprocessed, whereas now what you buy in your once-a-week shopping trip is processed— with most of the good removed from it. The simpler the food, the better we do.

I'm going to teach you about those foods that give you maximum energy with minimum effort. Freshness of course is an essential. Shop daily at the produce sec-tion of your own supermarket (better yet, do you still have an old-fashioned greengrocer?), pick up your dairy items, and assess the meat, poultry, and fish counter. Dine on what is freshest and best that day, not what you read about in some diet plan or other.

Buy just the appropriate amount for the precise number of people you will be feeding in your household. With your daily calendar in your hand, marked with the meals eaten in and the meals out, you will no longer emerge from the supermarket with the overload carried out by so many people who needlessly are weighing down their mind/body and their life.

One of the most pleasing secrets I can pass on to you is that it takes one-third or one-fourth less time to prepare food when you're cooking for the actual needs of your own life—and not for leftovers or the refrigerator or the garbage disposal. If you require four carrots, buy and cook four, not eight. If you're baking potatoes, think about the people who will be eating them: for this family member a small potato, for that one a larger potato. You'll begin to understand that we should eat according to the size we are and want to become. At all times the appropriate amount is very apparent.

AN INVITATION TO THE GOOD LIFE ONE DAY AT A TIME

The returning Golden Door guest (with rare exceptions, each and every guest returns) comes for the renewing and recharging that are part of a week devoted to listening to one's self and correctly zeroing in on the interpretation of one's own inner messages. It's wonderfully gratifying for me to hear these guests talk. These are people who have resolved their onetime dilemma about how and when to exercise, how and what to eat. And they know all about the why. Now, with the greatest joy, they are discovering new dimensions to their mind/body connection. They have chosen to become the drivers in their lives rather than the passengers. So will you.

Now, open your Golden Door. Begin.

Be practical. Don't bind yourself to a do-or-die approach. When you set yourself a modest goal at first, and reach it, and then set a more difficult one and reach that too, you're in training for success.

The Golden Door experiences involve these four parts of life and the proper balance between them all:

1. Movement—the essence of life
2. Relaxation—the creative conversion of stress
3. Nutrition—fuel for living completely and relaxing wholly
4. Joy—food for your many-dimensional spirit

1. Movement is the touchstone of health. Ancient man moved from dawn till dusk just to gather sufficient food to survive. Our survival is still predicated upon daily, extensive, variegated movement. The unextended body is the unlived-in body, the unlived-in life.

2. Relaxation, at the opposite end of the spectrum, is no less important. A healthy body cannot be chronically contracted, pent-up, and pinched. It must be shown how to stretch and relax and how to know the joy of being still. One can have proper relaxation only when it has been preceded by vigorous physical movement. You've read a lot of recent literature about stress reduction through exercise. It's all true. What are the alternatives? Pep pills, depressants, tranquilizers, stimulants, and other bad-trip drugs. Exercise is the valid antidote to negative stress. (Not all stress is avoidable or bad for you. A certain amount is necessary to existence. Stress intelligently and carefully applied can even be euphoric.)

FOR THE WOULD-BE RELAXER, SOMETIMES STOLEN MINUTES ARE SWEETEST

Another way to relax is simply to call time totally out. Take five or take ten, and take them and yourself far away from stressful situations. Impossible at home? Pull over to the side of the road when you are driving along a pleasant stretch. Skip the coffee portion of your coffee break at work. What do you do with your stolen five or ten minutes? Absolutely nothing. Just savor a few minutes alone. Don't think. Feel. Let your serenity become almost a tangible thing. How many times do you dutifully, reluctantly tear yourself away from a temptingly lovely scene? "I'd love to stay but I can't take the time" is your apologia. Stay. Take the time, if only five minutes. Let the moment fill you completely.

3. Nutrition is an elementary need. It truly is our fuel for both physical well-being and emotional health. Calories count—but far more important is the satisfaction your food gives you. A diet that deprives you of the pleasures of food cheats you of a valuable, even critical part of your life. You are the sum total of what you eat.

4. Joy is the invisible and irreplaceable ingredient of true health. Joy is the inevitable by-product of true oneness of body and spirit, that quality which when infused into your private world helps you to move up from the drab and commonplace and elevates any mere existence into consummate living.

GOOD HEALTH IS YOUR BIRTHRIGHT. RIGHT?

Don't sell yourself short as you make your future projections. Good health is not a privilege reserved for a few. To achieve it you merely need to reactivate an option you've held all along but haven't been *exercising*. Achieving a level of vibrant fitness is mostly a matter of letting your body enjoy itself.

And that also explains why this is not a diet book. In fact, it's an anti-diet book. The first three letters of the word "diet" tell the story all too well. To most people diets are a form of emotional suicide. I am writing about life enhancement.

ENJOY . . . ENJOY . . .

Most health regimens fail because they lack the element of enjoyment, and consequently they cannot be integrated into real life. They cause a little flurry and then burn out their converts, some with food deprivation, others with boring calisthenics, and all with overwhelming invitations to guilt. Astoundingly, they ignore the principle that only your increasingly robust enjoyment of life—not a weight chart, not a gym routine, not an improved pulse rate—can keep you going.

That is why the Golden Door approach has nothing to do with food deprivation, calisthenics, or guilt. Food is both pleasure and friend, and I mean to help you enhance that friendship. Exercise can be a bore; therefore I must make it irresistible.

Let me show you how to mine the full value from the calorie and also from the *psychological* calorie. Let me tell you how to extract every iota of benefit from movement and exercise. The first isn't fattening, the second involves no special effort. Yet you can double your pleasure, double your fun.

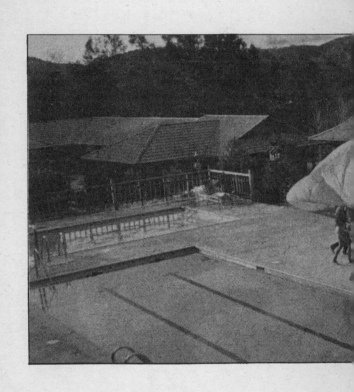

CHAPTER II

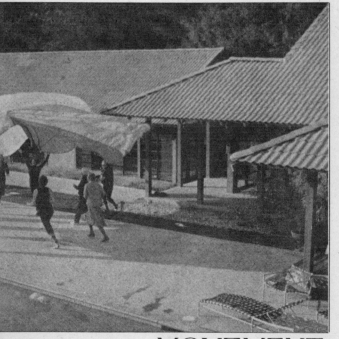

MOVEMENT:
THE DELIGHTS OF
PHYSICAL ACTIVITY

If you were to write down all of your physical activities every day for a week, I could guess your age. Everybody has a perceptible movement pattern, and most people over twenty-five are movement-starved.

Age is nearly always signaled by decreasing circles of movement. A young person moves in ever-widening circles. But then, there comes a time when you start saying, "It's too much trouble to go for a swim." Or, "Let's drive downtown. I don't feel like walking." Or, "I'd rather stay home." You move from the big house to the smaller one. Then to the ever-so-small and convenient condominium. As it becomes more and more restricted, life dwindles away bit by bit, and you put yourself into a box nature never intended for you.

Youth and beauty are always associated with kinetic behavior. Since the quality of your life depends upon your vitality, you must accept the fact that vitality comes from movement more than from any other single source. No matter what your age, you can reverse time's trend by moving more.

Are you worrying that exertion might be harmful? If you're a stranger to exercise, have a family history of heart ailments, are obese, smoke heavily, live on junk foods, or, in general, have a funky body, then do see a physician, preferably one who specializes in sports medicine.

Dr. Per Olof Astrand, a well-known exercise physiologist of the Swedish College of Physical Education, says, "As a general rule, moderate activity is less harmful to the healthy person than inactivity. A medical examination is more urgent for those who plan to stay inactive."

To an amazing extent, it turns out that the greater the amount of movement you exact from your body, the firmer its sense of health and well-being. Nor is this illusory. The systems of the body need work in order to stay strong and elastic. In fact, even patients with acute myocardial infarctions—for which prolonged bed rest was traditionally prescribed—are now finding themselves involved in carefully supervised physical exercise right there in the coronary-care unit, in a current experimental program. Doctors say this results in shortened hospitalization, enhanced cardiac function, and the elimination of a host of psychological and physical complications always provoked by enforced bed rest.

If you've ever broken an arm or a leg and been put in a cast, you know that immobility makes muscle tissue waste away rapidly. After the cast comes off, movement is tentative for a while, full of effort, and therefore tiring. That's a vivid analogy for what occurs very, very gradually when a body is allowed to slow down and become sedentary with age. It literally starts to wither away—although if the muscle tissue is replaced by fat the process sometimes is not visible from the outside.

What are your chances of remaining strong, vital, and

full of energy when you turn seventy? Pretty good, if that's how you are at thirty. A forty-year study by Henry S. Maas and Joseph A. Kuypers, researchers from the University of California, refutes the notion that you automatically are condemned to enfeeblement as you age. They discovered, among other things, that "Old age merely continued what earlier years had launched." But don't interpret this to mean that it's too late to reverse a negative trend. Exercise, slowly, carefully, and intelligently begun now, can help your bones absorb calcium, and keep you fairly erect and intact even when you're elderly. Better to get into the habit at least by your forties or fifties. But exercise expert Bonnie Prudden believes that being over fifty-five right now can be advantageous because you belong to a generation that walked to school, ran errands on foot, and probably pushed old-time nonelectric lawn mowers. She says the muscles you developed early on are still there and that you can still get into good shape within six to eight weeks—more quickly than many of today's lethargic teenagers could hope to do.

YOUR BUILT-IN YOUTH PRESERVER

Fortunately, you have within your body one miraculous part, invisible and indivisible, which has the capability to pull you out of trouble and forestall senescence. All is not lost. You still can reactivate your built-in youth preserver. That resource is the circulatory system.

Since your heart is a muscle, exercise affects it like any other muscle that can improve and grow stronger. The improved heart muscle pumps more blood with each stroke and beats fewer times per minute. Even during exercise (or under the stress of anger or anxiety), the conditioned heart doesn't beat as rapidly as the heart that's been weakened by indolence. It returns to its "resting" rate sooner. It stands to reason that if you can strengthen your heart through saving it thousands of beats, by the time you're sixty it will show less wear and tear than if you had neglected it.

The following is a brief summary intended to encapsulate the gist of what so many medical journals report:

Regular exercise enables you to recover more quickly from stress. After a good exercise workout your bodily functions won't return at once to their poor pre-exercise level. For a while you'll continue to breathe more efficiently, your oxygen level will remain high, and you'll burn fat more steadily.

YOUR DYNAMIC DUO

At the Golden Door we believe that the cardiovascular system is inseparable from the pulmonary system, i.e., heart and blood vessels and lungs. Our exercises are designed to give equal emphasis to both systems, whereas most other exercise regimens ignore this relationship. Again, I'll state the case very simply: The heart and the lungs are inextricably bound in constant interplay; one cannot function effectively without the other. The oxygen your circulating blood carries is obtained through the lungs. Your heart circulates the blood through your lungs each time it goes through that familiar two-phase cycle of pump-rest, pump-rest. When your heart contracts, it forces blood through those miles of blood vessels. The contraction is followed by a rest period, and during this rest your blood fills your heart with just the right amount to be pumped out again in the next contraction. During exercise more blood than usual comes into the heart, which is stretched more; it then contracts more vigorously and pumps out more blood than before. This is the heart's intrinsic way of exercising its muscle.

Here is where the lungs come into play. The lungs are located within the rib cage; this chamber develops a negative pressure whenever you take in a really deep breath. The normal chest cage and lungs never have inside pressure equal to outside pressure. This negative pressure during inspiration is one of the factors helping to bring the blood back to the heart. The deeper the breath you inhale, the more negative pressure is created and the more blood comes back to your heart.

During exercise, this extraordinary coordination between your lungs and your heart becomes even more important. Because of the demands of tissue—such as those of your leg muscles when you run, or your diaphragm when you run—your requirement for oxygen and nutrients there is so much greater. More blood has to be pumped to the tissue.

AND YET YOUR HEART
NEVER HAS JET LAG

The heart's 100,000 beats every twenty-four hours are sufficient to move over 4,000 (theoretical) gallons of blood through the lungs and on into 60,000 (actual figure) miles of blood vessels. The heart's only rest is a fractional second between beats. The heart has no rear end to sit upon.

The straightest route to cardiovascular/pulmonary health is to exercise for recreation and re-creation. Choose an exercise that gives you pleasure, increases your heart and respiratory rates, and causes a welcome sense of fatigue while reducing tension. With regular exercise you will recover more quickly from stress than you would if your heart weren't pumping so efficiently. Best of all, after a good workout your bodily functions won't return at once to poor pre-exercise levels.

And, if you continue to keep all systems open and functioning at full capacity, your looks will reflect the vivacity you feel.

WE WEREN'T BUILT TO SIT STILL

Imagine you're an apprentice historian in some distant millennium. Without any other frame of reference you are handed a microfilm of a number of ancient periodicals from a country called the United States of America, circa A.D. 1970–1980. Your assignment: Analyze the country's social structure.

Here's what you very well might write:

All riches and honors were reserved for a privileged few, called sports superstars. These individuals were treated like demigods, and great crowds gathered to cheer them in various reproductions of the Circus Maximus.

An epidemic of heart disease was sweeping the land. Medical knowledge, although crude, already had established the heart's need for exercise. Tragically, only a few were able to profit from this scientific breakthrough.

Among the citizenry a campaign had begun to claim the right to exercise in order to prolong life. But these efforts were generally spasmodic and not well organized.

The condition of the majority of the people was pathetic. At work they were cruelly confined indoors and at the end of each day's toil they were sequestered in cells from which they seldom moved.

Most fiendish of all was the practice of televising for these unfortunates scene after scene of those life-giving activities in which they were forbidden to participate.

Does that really sound so absurd?

ARMCHAIR ATHLETES
DON'T RUN UP ANY POINTS

Too many people today experience the complete, joyous, multidimensional world of sports activity vicariously only through television, radio, and newspapers. To this they so easily could be adding a whole rainbow spectrum of body experience that would transform their lives.

Let me be very specific about all the rewards of exercise. You can expect payoff in the way of:

1. Psychological bonuses
2. Exorcising of tension and stress
3. Eating without stringent diets

Exercise makes you feel competent, powerful, and proud. As your self-esteem increases, you will find a parallel effect on your total life-style.

EXERCISE—NOT AN ONUS
BUT A BONUS

Taking the initiative in the matter of body movement is certain to make you feel like a winner. Exercise is the surest antidote to the poisonous miasma of mental depression, which cannot coexist with optimal physiological/psychological well-being. If you feel mental distress, and are dreading decisions, it is crucial that you avoid inertia. Move affirmatively. Whenever you feel low, get high on movement. Research conducted in numerous hospitals with drug addicts and schizophrenics showed lasting improvement through marathon running—reuniting and restructuring the balance of mind and body. Many tests over the past years indicate that, after a vigorous forty-minute workout, the physiological benefits are measurable—and so is the high, which remains with you on a decreasing scale for the next six hours.

PSYCHING OUT THE
BREATH OF LIFE

In 1970 I was a guinea pig in an early biofeedback experimentation program with Dr. Barbara Brown, renowned authority and author of *New Mind, New Body.* During those months I was hypersensitized to the relationship of mind and body, and my experiences blossomed into new insights. This was my most exciting discovery: I found that through manipulating my breathing I could also manipulate my brain waves, and I realized that breathing is a major factor in altering our states of consciousness. Therefore I believe that exercise, with its singular effect on breathing, can achieve this.

In many forms of meditation and prayer, the ritual establishes a specific, continuous breathing pattern— the Arab answering the call of his muezzin, the Jew wrapped in his prayer shawl, and the Catholic saying his beads. Sleep also has its own special breathing pattern, and ecstasy is frequently described as "breath-less."

What I largely intuited then has now been confirmed in *Some Psychological Effects of Physical Conditioning*, a treatise by Dr. Thaddeus Kostrubala. This study describes an altered state of consciousness rich with intellectual associations, which are experienced as insights, and a shift in perception as the visual experience assumes a unique aesthetic importance.

WHEN TO DO YOUR NUMBER

Early in 1975 I had the good fortune of meeting Dr. Kostrubala. For nineteen months he both participated in a running program and recorded his observations in his book, *The Joy of Running*. The goal of the program was to run nonstop for from forty to sixty minutes, three times a week, at 75 percent of one's maximum cardiac output. To quote from his study:

> It appears that the physical running aspects of the program act as a catalyst upon the established life patterns of the individuals . . . there are distinct psychologic changes which occur when physiologic improvement takes place . . . decreased depression, decreased irritability and an increasing sense of confidence and well-being . . . a reawakening of libidinal energy . . . euphoria . . . the feeling of increased energy after the exercise period.

The very time of day causes exercise's psychological bonuses to vary. I advocate a good 60 minutes daily, distributed according to the exigencies of your present-day life. Most people find 30 minutes in the morning, 10 at high noon, and 20 in the late day a feasible schedule. You may twist the schedule around to 40-10-10. However you slice it, the crucial consideration is that you must have at least one 20-minute period of continuous stressful exercise if you are to build your cardiovascular and pulmonary strength.

Personally, I walk/run for a full hour in the morning,

7:30 to 8:30, plus five minutes of exercise (stretching and jump-rope) before lunch and repeated as I change before preparing dinner. This schedule works best for me, since I seem to get busier as the day proceeds. Whatever works for you is the best schedule of all.

A PAYOFF IN TURN-ONS

If you allow yourself 30 minutes or more in the morning, you will do everything that day with greater efficiency and greater joy because you have set out with a measurable physiologic high. And because you set a goal and carried it out with comparative ease, you will find you have a new habit of successful goal-setting.

Exercise, says sports-medicine authority Dr. Gabe Mirkin, "curbs hunger. When you exercise, fat is released into your bloodstream and your blood-sugar level doesn't drop. And low blood sugar is the single most important stimulus to make you hungry. So when people exercise, they are likely to eat less."

But when women were polled about the rewards of strenuous exercise, they were most enthusiastic about changes in their emotional life. They credited exercise with everything from relieving their depressions and anxieties to giving them increased confidence, better social relations, and an improved self-image.

Running teacher Roger Eischens was quoted with this perceptive analysis: "The thing that makes people feel good is the actual feedback from the muscles, the tissues, the heart, and the lungs. It tells them they're alive."

YOUR DAILY ENERGY IS ON
A DOWNHILL COURSE.
LEARN HOW TO PICK IT UP.

Our natural energy is on a steady downward slide between eight A.M. and noon. The white wine or martini at lunch only accelerates the slide. But noontime exercise will return you to your desk or to your routine

---

at home with your energy curve pumped back up to the nine–ten-A.M. level. The change of pace and the relaxation that are the by-products of an exercise break will see you through a moderate-sized lunch because you won't be looking to food to give you all your strokes. If you have a weight-loss goal, you will find a small yogurt, nuts, and fruit lunch satisfactory.

HOW TO EXORCISE
TENSION AND STRESS

Several years ago we at the Golden Door conducted a private poll of nearly a thousand supposedly healthy upper-income people in the Southwestern United States. The large response to the poll was surprising, and so were the findings concerning tension. An overwhelming number of men and women of all ages replied that, although they slept soundly all night, every night, they awakened feeling physically tired. Given the busy social lives and heavy civic and business commitments of these people, as a nonprofessional analyst I found it simple to conclude that, while their minds were continually engaged throughout the day, their bodies remained inactive. They went to bed with minds weary from use but with bodies still charged up and tense—no chance to reach the sweet mind-body balance so necessary for the sort of sleep that renews. Of course I'm not the only one who has pondered this phenomenon.

GET IN SYNC OR
BE OUT OF THE SWIM

What a pity that using your head means using your rear as well. No wonder educational institutions talk about seats of learning. The more hours your mind moves, or simply worries and fidgets around, the more hours you sit. As you rise from your desk, stretch, and yawn at the end of the day, a great chasm yawns between body and mind. You are entirely out of sync. The only way to put it all together is to do just that. As you run, walk, bicycle, whatever, you retune your body and restore it to synchronization. A number of scientists who have been comparing exercise with such tranquilizers as meprobamate and alcohol say exercise wins every time. A session of vigorous movement at the end of working hours is a marvelous way to rid yourself of pent-up emotions. As you move, you can give expression to all the things you couldn't say during the day. One reason tennis has become so widely and wildly popular is that as you hit the ball you can actually holler "Go to hell!" or whatever you've been bursting to unburden yourself of. And even the exercise of brisk walking gives you a chance to transform aggressions and tensions into creative energy.

Unrelieved stress is the villain. Its relief can best be accomplished through aggressive movement. Once you know ways to counter tension, you needn't worry so much about high-stress situations. When the crisis moment is past, you'll at once readjust and transmit peace hosannas to all the parts of your body, because you will have learned how to coexist comfortably with stress. Rabindranath Tagore said it well: "Rest belongs to the work as the eyelids to the eyes."

I DON'T ASK YOU
TO STRING ALONG WITH
A STRINGENT DIET

Emphasis will go where it belongs, on a truly sensible, well-balanced food plan incorporating the great variety of natural foodstuffs providing the minerals, vitamins, amino acids, etc., that are required if we are to maintain the body's health. If your life-style is stressful, or if you have quite a lot of weight to lose, then plan for weight loss on alternate months. Four weeks on our food plan will assure a slow, steady weight loss. Then supplement your food plan each day with natural whole-grain dishes to convert to a healthful maintenance diet.

We will, together, create a workable exercise program to burn up the stored energy/fuel/food rather than sentence you to another semistarvation regime. You do not need to lose your health while you lose weight. Exercise allows you to enjoy your food more and also entitles you to more food to enjoy. You quite simply get to eat more than you would if you were inactive. According to metabolic law, you must balance food taken in with energy expended. So won't it be enough just to diet? Not only are most "wonder diets" masochistic, unsatisfying, and impermanent even in their superficial results, they really aren't good for you. On a strict, no-exercise diet you may be losing weight by burning off fat together with parts of your precious "lean body mass"—muscle and other nonfat tissue.

MAKE IT EASY ON YOURSELF

You may not even need to lose as much weight as you think. A taut body can look and feel pounds lighter. To achieve this is the main thrust of the exercise program at the Golden Door.

Therefore, abandon any fad diet you may be on and substitute common sense. Learn sensible eating, and then let exercise multiply its effects. The result: a trim figure and a healthy glow to show it off.

CALORIES TO BURN

You must learn how to fine-tune your system by correlating a day's activities with the size of your meals. To help you with beauty's new math, Frank Konishi, Professor of Nutrition at Southern Illinois University, has devised a common-sense tool. His book, *Exercise Equivalents of Foods,* contains the basic information for honing down to a prettier, skinnier, more vivid You.

The Konishi book tells you how many calories are lurking within almost every kind of food imaginable. Then it lists the corresponding number of minutes of exercise—whether walking, bicycling, stepping, swimming, or jogging—you would have to put forth to burn off the calories in each food serving. Should you wish to know how many days will be required to lose a certain number of pounds, with a particular combination of calorie reduction and exercise, the book also has tables for that. Keep this little book handy in your kitchen. It can graphically and indelibly impress upon you the connection between the (food) energy input and (exercise) energy output. If you can't find the title in your bookstore, ask them to order it from Southern Illinois University Press, Carbondale, Illinois.

Let me qualify the following chart by saying that *you* will probably make the proportion of calories-to-minutes-of-exercise somewhat variable. You create the variability by

    1. your size
    2. how you seize upon the activity at hand
       (be vigorous, and all the figures will
       balance out in your favor)

BODY SENSE

The French use an apt phrase, *élan vital,* to express lithe, jaunty, vigorous spirits. It describes very well the inner light that emerges when people adhere to a creative exercise plan. And you don't have to go to the Golden Door to find your body sense.

The first two articles I did for *Vogue* magazine about a decade ago were concerned mostly with rope-skipping and my fondness for it, which the editor thought very novel of me. Nobody had considered the jump rope for years, outside of fighters in training. "Jumping is a natural, undisciplined exertion," I wrote in *Vogue.* "It appeals to the child in us, and it enables us to use that child as an ally. . . . Jumping in bare feet seems to help. . . . And just try jumping with poor posture. . . .

"A jump rope happens to be my favorite route to huff-and-puff. I keep one in my car, my office, my briefcase, and my bedroom. It nimbles legs, upper arms, and torso, and builds up posture and stamina. Buy good solid jump rope from a sporting-goods store, not the lightweight variety sold in toy shops. Increase your

MINUTES REQUIRED AT THE EXERCISES LISTED TO EXPEND CALORIES IN THE FOODS

FOOD	CALORIES	ACTIVITY					
		Walking Minutes	Stepping Minutes	Bicycling Minutes	Jogging Minutes	Swimming Minutes
Apple, 1 medium	87	17	12	11	9	8
Bacon, crisp, 2 slices	96	19	13	12	10	9
Banana, 1 medium	127	24	17	16	13	11
Beans, green, ½ cup cooked	15	3	2	2	2	1
Beer, 8-ounce glass	115	22	15	14	12	10
Bread and butter, 1 slice	96	18	13	12	10	9
Cake, white layer, 1/16 of 9" cake	250	48	33	31	25	22
Carrot, raw, 1 large	42	8	6	5	4	4
Cereal, dry, 1 cup, with milk and sugar	212	41	28	26	21	19
Cheese, American, 1-ounce slice	112	22	15	14	11	10
Cheese, cottage, 1 rounded tablespoon	30	6	4	4	3	3

Food					
Chicken, fried, ½ breast	232	45	31	28	23	21
Chicken, TV dinner	542	104	72	66	54	48
Cola beverage, 8-ounce glass	105	20	14	13	11	9
Cookie, chocolate-chip, 1 average	50	10	7	6	5	5
Cookie, vanilla-wafer, 1 average	15	3	2	2	2	1
Doughnut, 1 average	125	24	17	15	13	11
Egg, boiled or poached, 1 medium	78	15	10	10	8	7
Egg, fried or scrambled, 1 medium	108	21	14	13	11	10
French dressing, 1 tablespoon	57	11	8	7	6	5
Gelatin, with cream, 1 serving	117	23	16	14	12	10
Halibut, broiled, 1 serving	214	41	28	26	21	19
Ham, fresh, 2 slices cooked	254	49	34	31	25	23
Ice cream, ⅔ cup	186	36	25	23	19	17
Ice-cream soda, 1 regular	255	49	34	31	26	23
Ice milk, ⅔ cup	137	26	18	17	14	12
Malted milk, 8-ounce glass	500	96	67	61	50	45

FOOD	CALORIES	ACTIVITY				
Mayonnaise, 1 tablespoon	100	19	13	12	10	9
Milk, skim, 8-ounce glass	88	17	12	11	9	8
Milk, whole, 8-ounce glass	160	36	21	20	16	14
Milk shake, 8-ounce glass	420	81	56	51	42	38
Orange, 1 medium	73	14	10	9	7	7
Orange juice, 4-ounce glass	54	10	7	7	5	5
Pancake, 1, with 2 tablespoons syrup	204	39	27	25	20	18
Peach, 1 medium	38	7	5	5	4	3
Peach shortcake, 1 biscuit and 1 peach	266	51	35	32	27	24
Peas, green, ½ cup cooked	58	11	8	7	6	5
Pie, fruit, ⅙ of 9" pie	400	77	53	49	40	36
Pie, pecan, ⅙ of 9" pie	670	129	89	82	67	60
Pizza, cheese, ⅛ of 14" pie	185	36	25	23	19	17
Pork chop, 6 ounces raw	314	60	42	38	31	28
Potato chips, five 2" chips	54	10	7	7	5	5
Club (bacon, chicken, tomato) Sandwiches	590	114	78	72	59	53

Hamburger	350	67	47	43	35	31
Roast beef with gravy	430	83	57	52	43	38
Tuna salad	278	54	37	34	28	25
Sherbet, orange, ⅔ cup	120	23	16	15	12	11
Shrimp, French-fried, 3½ ounces	225	43	30	27	23	20
Spaghetti, meat sauce, 1 serving	396	76	53	48	40	35
Steak, T-bone, ½ pound raw	235	45	31	29	24	21

ENERGY COST FOR 154-POUND INDIVIDUAL, 5'9" TALL.
If you weigh less, your caloric "costs" may be lower.
WALKING briskly at 3.5 to 4 miles per hour on the average consumes 5.2 calories per minute.
STEPPING 25 up and down steps per minute facing in the same direction consumes an average of 7.5 calories per minute.
BICYCLING consumes around 8.2 calories per minute.
JOGGING alternated with walking (5 minutes each jogging, walking, jogging, etc.) consumes around 10 calories per minute.
SWIMMING with average skill consumes approximately 11.2 calories per minute.

ADAPTED FROM "EXERCISE EQUIVALENTS OF FOOD," BY FRANK KONISHI, PH.D., SOUTHERN ILLINOIS UNIVERSITY PRESS (1973). USED BY PERMISSION OF *FAMILY CIRCLE MAGAZINE*.

quota of jumps and the speed with which you turn the rope with each two-minute session. . . . When to exercise? Just before meals. Before breakfast to oil away wake-up stiffness. Before lunch and dinner to soothe tensions that build up over hours of busy-ness. Like a well-balanced mainspring, exercise both winds and unwinds, and is great before you need to make an earthshaking appearance or before you embark on a dazzling evening.''

I think I touched off an industry. People of all ages are jumping these days, and some of them are writing books on the subject. One of these books has researched all the rhymes children used to recite while skipping. They're fun to recall, and it really was as a fun substitute for run/jog that I started packing my jump rope around in the first place. Jumping too is being examined as a cardiovascular exercise. Some claim 10 minutes of rope work is worth 30 minutes of roadwork, but at the same time warn that strenuous jumping can be hard on the heart.

YOUR FITNESS—JUST A HOP, SKIP, AND A JUMP AWAY

To determine the right length for your jump rope, step on it at midpoint. Either end should reach your underarms, and if it hits the floor when you jump, it is probably in need of shortening. If you're not jumping indoors on well-carpeted floors, you'll need jogging shoes or other footwear with cushioned soles; and comfortable clothing of course. As with other serious exercise, start off with a few simple warm-ups, such as our Pre-Anything Exercises (pages 105–81). If you're not in the peak of condition, it will be better to run over the rope with one foot after the other rather than to land simultaneously on the soles of both feet. And nothing is gained by jumping too high.

But don't leap into jumping if you have a bad back! (At the Golden Door, we concentrate on back-babying. That's how the stretching and back-strengthening Pre-Anything Exercises developed.)

EVERY DAY IS MOVING DAY

I prefer jumping rope as an easy introduction to the joys of physical activity. As you recognize how integral movement is to the quality of a joyous life, you're going to become more and more aware of your needs for movement. A body grows to rely on its daily movement-nourishment. Once revved up, you may note how easily you feel stifled by lack of fresh air or lack of moving around. You'll be annoyed by long periods of inactivity and will want to follow them with a brisk walk, swim, or jog. Or with the ubiquitous jump rope.

You can even turn any kind of housework into body-sculpturing exercise. Play rhythmic music while you work. Open the windows and let fresh air fill your lungs. Alternate bending-over chores with jobs that require stretching, such as washing walls.

Once you have made what I call body sense a part of your repertoire for living, you'll want to preserve its continuity, for you will find the urge to exercise (body sense) as basic an urge as appetite or thirst.

VERY EASY DOES IT!

But if you *do* fall into the trap of a long period of enforced idleness once you're an exercise regular, remember to ease yourself back into your routine, slowly.

When I was fifty I was a June bride. On our honeymoon we traveled 25,000 miles. It was an in-and-out-of-planes-cars-and-hotels month. Then, at last, we were home. To eradicate those long periods of being compressed into a tight capsule, I chose to spend my recovery day on the beach with a younger friend. We arrived mid-morning, strolled for hours along the sands, chased sand crabs and sandpipers, napped, then walked again. In the evening our husbands joined us. After picnicking we ran along the shore. At last I had stretched! At last I had breathed fully!

The next morning, I couldn't get out of bed. I had developed bursitis of the knee—which made me more than usually aware of my body, and demonstrated how easy it is to overdo.

Yes, I had behaved as gauchely as any of my most chairbound guests who, adjusting to a spa program for the first time, try too hard to catch up on activity long missed. My only excuse is that I overreacted to what I believe is a natural "movement instinct." Slothfulness makes me feel imprisoned, and a day without any real movement seems like a day in jail.

Your common sense already has persuaded you that there's no quickie approach to the joys of physical activity. Fitness depends upon fidelity to a continuing program. Exercise cannot be stored. There is a potent incentive to spur you to daily activity: the high you sustain because you now respect your ability to control your own destiny.

DAWN MAN WAS BORN WITH GET UP AND GO

For primitive man, there was no question of deliberating these pros and cons of movement, nor for our forebears of one hundred or even fifty years ago. If they were to eat, they had to move. Now our environment has changed, but our bodies remain similar to those pictured in prehistoric cave drawings.

What a pity we of today have to wait till we're adults before realizing how exercise can enrich our lives. I recall a junior-high physical-education instructor who blew a whistle frequently and bounced a volleyball while shouting, "Okay! Everybody out on the playground!" But at no point were we students taught the optimum exertion we need to keep in trim. Nor have my children learned it in their school. My dream is to see training for living with one's body included as a required course in physical education. The sooner we begin to understand the basics of good health, the better we all will be, both as individuals and as a nation.

THE TOOTH FAIRY
HAS HAD GOOD P.R.

On the other hand, children in this country are bombarded with information about their teeth. A study once proved it takes the average girl child till age eight, and a boy till twelve, to make toothbrushing automatic. As a result, whenever we walk into the bathroom we don't have to dawdle about and run through what we can remember about dental care. We just reach for the toothbrush without delay. Behind that reflex is a lot of nagging by parents, filmstrips in school, cards from the dentist that told you to come in and pick out a gift—and, if all else failed, there was the immediacy of a toothache and a drill-wielding dentist saying, "See? See what happens when you don't brush?"

Dental associations have done such a first-class job of public information that it's difficult to grow up in America and not know the fundamentals of home dental care.

OUR KIDS AREN'T GETTING
THE WORD ABOUT THEIR
FITNESS FAIRY GODMOTHER

Our sense of priorities needs modifying. After all, you can live without a single tooth in your head and buy a fair manmade set, but you cannot buy a brand new and satisfactory heart. I only wish heart associations could begin as early to broadcast their message. They might avert what's been called the twentieth-century epidemic: coronary disease. Unfortunately it is caused by no single, easily pinpointed factor. But topping the treacherous list of likely causes of heart degeneration is our sedentary life-style.

Ideally, we would have learned healthy movement habits in childhood. Instead, schools promote immobility. As babies and toddlers we were once lively as puppy dogs. But today the first thing we do is to send the child off to preschool, so he will learn to sit still and pay attention. The teacher plays a tune on the piano while the children walk about the room. When the music stops, each child sits on a colored dot. It is the preschool's prime achievement. (Of course, the teacher receives an assist from the thousands of hours* which even a three-year-old has already rolled up on the TV log—a practice which like the reliance on junk food has led to the alarming rising trend toward obesity among U.S. children.)

Soon the child learns to grit his teeth and sit quietly throughout the entire school day—something that cannot be taught to even the most well-bred chimpanzee.

HOW TO PLAN YOUR
PHYSICAL ACTIVITY

"You're in good shape for a man who spends his time behind the desk," I said one day to a Golden Door guest who was a member of the President's Cabinet.

"Well," he said, "before I started coming to the Golden Door, exercise was always a catch-as-catch-can proposition. I would play golf occasionally, swim when I could, walk once in a while.

"But at the Door I learned the value of regularity, and particularly the value of wake-up exercise. At home I spend thirty minutes in the morning, seven days a week, right after getting out of bed, in my bedroom with the television news on. For the first ten minutes I'm on my stationary bicycle, and for the next twenty I do various exercises I learned in the wake-up session that starts the day here at the Golden Door—they follow a fluid pattern from one to the next, some standing up and some on the floor.

"It's now such a habit that if I miss the morning exercises because of travel or tight scheduling of some sort, I don't feel right. I feel sluggish. Since I don't take the

*Owing to the national habit of employing the TV set as a babysitter, no less a source than a 1974 Nielsen survey estimated that the average U.S. three-year-old puts in an average of 30 hours a week television viewing.

bicycle along when I travel, I do some extra running in my hotel room—again, while watching TV news to relieve the monotony of solo exercising."

IN YOUR OWN TIME, IN YOUR OWN STYLE

I quote this conversation to illustrate what I always tell my guests about exercise: "Although I go to some trouble to give you guidelines for the kind of exercising I hope will be ideal for you, *I don't care how you do it, as long as you do it.*" Think of all the most efficacious exercise movements as a smorgasbord. After a little sampling you're sure to find something you want to stay with.

Best of all, try to settle on exercise that's both *isotonic* and *aerobic.*

An isotonic exercise is one that involves rhythmic, repetitive tensing and relaxing of muscles: dancing, bicycling, walking, swimming, rowing, skipping rope, working out on a mat, jogging on a mini-trampoline, and so forth. The repeated squeezing of the muscles helps the blood flow and promotes cardiovascular pulmonary fitness.

An aerobic exercise is one that you can continue to perform for more than a few minutes, with oxygen being supplied to the exercising muscles all during that time. Sprinting, for example, is not aerobic because the average person can't run full blast for more than a few seconds.

PICK YOUR FAVORITES. You're going to be the final judge of what you and your body find likable. Together, we'll create for you a supple, bend-to-your-whim, workable schedule. The result will be a fresh pattern of movement planned especially for you and your individual life. The most wonder-working fitness trick is to make every day's physical activity into a reflex, so automatic it becomes a habit, and to smoothly fit it into its proper, most advantageous time slot.

NATURE—
THE FORCE IS WITH YOU

As we traverse these pages, I will move from the practical to the theoretic, the physiologic to the psychologic. There is an added and effortless plus when your mind recognizes its involvement with your body, as both feel their oneness with the moving currents of nature that lie within us, as surely as within any beast, tree, or stream.

Begin the day deeply within your body. Spend a few moments in bed feeling your body, tense, relax, tense again, relax. Become aware of this—your real home. Smile, take a deep breath. Feel it. And most of all, like yourself. And remember—you're not taking just your head out of bed.

Occasionally play the ancestor game. Put yourself in the position of one of your own forebears—100, 500, or 1,000 years ago. Imagine him awaking in a farmer's cot. Your day will stretch through long hours, but he cannot dawdle considering his options. If he is going to eat, he will have to move. No one to coax him, to imply how much fun it will be to milk ten cows before breakfast, how grand to fell trees, or to hoe, or weed the cotton. So up, up, and away.

To ensure our survival, nature fashioned us for movement. We either move toward life or away from it. That is our only real option.

Cher quickly discovered how much closer to nature you feel when you run out to meet it at the birth of day. "I love the Golden Door because it has everything," she says. "But above all it has that heavenly path for the early-morning uphill walk.

"When I first spent two weeks at the Door, I was building a new house. I had to hurry home to see if I could have my own morning-walk path out back. I could. I have. And I use it."

YOUR GOLDEN DOOR PLAN

1. BEGIN THE DAY WITH A TOE-TWISTER. Do this even before you get your head together: While half-awake and vulnerable to impressions, keep your eyes closed and take a deep breath. Let it out. Take another, and let it halfway out.

Then follow the lead of Ruth West, who has written many books on food and health, and is one of the most dynamic, slender, and stylish over-seventy women I've ever known. When Ruth wakes up in her New York apartment, she exercises in bed. "That's something I learned at the Golden Door," she told me.

> Exercises before I get up are marvelous because I'm too lazy to do any other kind—when I first wake up, anyway. Later, I love to walk and dance and move around a lot. But here's what I do first thing in the morning: I start with twisting my toes, turning my feet around from the ankles. Then I splay them and stretch them out. I raise and lower my legs about ten times, slowly. The next thing is what you'd just do naturally. I extend each leg alternately and stretch my arms above my head. Then I get up.

Next, Ruth performs some stretching exercises which we'll come to in a moment. Also, I must tell you of one of her favorite ploys: she pays for tennis lessons in advance, in order to be committed to taking them. "But those first little stretching exercises in bed!" she exclaims. "I couldn't start the day without them."

2. THE NAKED TRUTH. The next thing you are to do is my own special secret for reminding yourself that you're about to begin another day of living for life. It will take you just two minutes every morning.

Stepping out of bed is a propitious time for imprinting your plans and intentions for the day. Use what once was called autosuggestion. Get out of bed and stand nude, with your eyes wide open, in front of a full-length mirror. You haven't yet put on your "character armor" for the day, so you can make a very candid inventory of yourself. Stand straight and still before the mirror. Experience your Self. During two minutes of stretching, pulling, reaching, warming-up exercises, gradually mold a vision of the person you wish to be. Reproduce that image in the mirror, and make sure it is a smiling one, eagerly anticipating the day and the pleasant surprises to be found in the hours to come.

Stretch each limb, one at a time, as a cat does upon waking. Rotate your head on your neck. Tuck in your chin. Elongate your spine. Stand tall. Shrug your shoulders back and forth, loosening your diaphragm and rib cage so you can feel your ribs floating high and free. Raise each knee and feel the contraction and relaxation pulse through your loins as you bring knee to chest. Then, standing with feet together, spread your toes and bounce on the balls of your feet.

At first, these two minutes in the morning will be a means of determining where you are. After a while you'll be using them to calculate where you want to go. And you'll become increasingly aware how productive just two well-applied minutes can be.

3. ONE STEP AT A TIME. You may have to make a few passes at settling on the program ideally suited to you. But do persist. Take things one step at a time, moving to a new goal a bit farther ahead each time you reach an older one. If you are young and very active, you may aspire to be able eventually to run a fast mile, or six miles, a mini-marathon, or even the big one—the marathon itself. Or you simply may want to acquire the ability to do your very first push-up. Or to touch your fingers to the floor. Or to lose two inches off your waistline.

Take inventory at the beginning of your program, then one month later, and thereafter at three-month intervals. Of course, you can check more frequently if you perform better on a shorter leash. Whatever works and will continue to work for you is your way to go.

Two methods I have found effective are:
  a. Tricks of a Ten-Percenter—for the person who already is fairly active
  b. Sixty Minutes of the Prime Time of Your Life

a. TRICKS OF A TEN-PERCENTER. If you're in your twenties or thirties and have one specific bulge you wish to erase, being a ten-percenter will probably suffice. Odds are high that you run and jump and dance and play often enough to keep your circulatory system perking. With just a bits-and-pieces exercise program, you soon will stand taller, be trimmer, and whip about with better muscle tone.

Ask yourself how you can slyly insert 10 percent more movement into all the normal activities of your day, adding just a little here and there. Park your car blocks away from your appointment and walk. Step off the elevator a few floors below the one you want and walk up the stairs. Remove all your extension phones.

The ten-percent route is a particularly good way to reach some of the parts of your body that tend to get lost and never receive any workouts: If tension localizes in your neck during the day, for example, you can use the wait at a stoplight to roll your head in a circle or do some loosening exercise you find relaxing.

On shorter errands, use a bicycle instead of a car. Park at the far end of the shopping center's lot. Carry your own groceries to your bike or car, or all the way home if you don't live too far away—a task you can lighten by shopping every day for crisp dewy-fresh foods instead of packing home a huge load once a week (see "Glorious Eating," page 241).

NEITHER RAIN, NOR SLEET, NOR . . .

Don't use unfavorable weather as an excuse to let down. If you can't pleasurably walk around outdoors, then push on to that gallery or museum show you've been wanting to drop in on.

At Christmas-time 1978, I spent a week in Aspen. The house I rented had a huge window wall overlooking the snow-covered road and fields, and as I sat re-reading the final draft of this book, it seemed as though it was just for my benefit that every fifteen or twenty minutes a jogger would run by. Dozens, of all ages, ran through the deep, soft snow and in spite of the 8,000-foot altitude. I felt so proud watching them, for I know that in my own small way, through the Ranch and the Golden Door, I have contributed to this phenomenon.

Snowbound? Hop on a stationary bicycle, the one absolutely indispensable item of exercise equipment in any household.

People in offices ought to replace the coffee break with a movement break. It's a change of pace your body silently craves, more than it wants a prune Danish, a cigarette, or coffee. So walk quickly around the block. Or jump rope through the building corridors (any glances that come your way will be ones of envy). Once you have begun to enjoy yourself, every activity at home or work will trigger some extra exercise idea. And you'll be in shape before you know it.

Single women who work are particularly subject to rainy-day blues if after five brings you home to a place that seems lonely because stormy weather is visible through the windowpanes. Be your own morale builder. Start the day wearing your brightest or newest outfit. You'll feel head and shoulders above all the people who use bad weather as an excuse for looking tacky. Plunge out and have your hair done on your lunch hour. Stop by the Y for a late-day exercise class, tension workout, or a swim. Take pleasure in yourself, and toward evening your refrigerator won't seem to light up with all the allure of the Blue Grotto.

b. SIXTY MINUTES OF THE PRIME TIME OF YOUR LIFE. It's my fervent belief that the basic requirement for your well-being and good looks is a daily hour of exercise. However, you might get by on forty minutes a day (but no less) at least three times a week. Try for five times, Monday through Friday, to allow some leeway for the occasional rainstorm or breakfast meeting—and if you can steal time from the weekend, so much the better.

Golden Door graduates return to their homes with an exercise plan that comes in two styles: one for the person who likes to complete most of a day's work before noon (I also recommend this as a solution for the hate-to-get-up type), and the other for the person who needs extra help in untwisting the knots at the end of the day. We all require some exercises for both getting up and getting down.

The Morning Pattern—Winding Up: Forty minutes of springy exercise and hard breathing, including a few minutes for warm-up and cool-down, as part of your breakfast time can point you toward a nice clear high. A brisk walk-jog is a joyous beginning. Or practice some of the exercises shown later in this book. Afterward, you'll absolutely float through the day. Then you'll require a refresher of ten minutes at noon and at least ten more minutes of exercise at twilight.

The Evening Pattern—Winding Down: The pattern for the evening person is the mirror opposite of the morning. If your day is taut with high-tension situations, you may have no trouble getting up for it but you will have trouble settling down later. The best way to approach such a day is to start before breakfast with twenty minutes of vigorous exercise. Then you get in a few licks during your ten minutes at noon. The important thirty-minute stint will come at twilight, before dinner. This is a life-saver, of particular importance whenever you've had a trying day which called up a lot of fight-or-flight reflexes to which you were unable to respond. Your ancestor, primitive man or woman, could run for dear life or stand up and fight for that life when very survival was threatened—thanks to the spurt of adrenaline with which nature empowers the muscles. Nature delivers adrenaline to you, too, without giving it any place to go. Civilized man, threatened, usually can neither fight nor run. Anger and resentment are held within, and tension with no place to go becomes hostile to the mind/body. The result is the tension headache, the heartburn, the ulcers, hemorrhoids, or the lower-back pain—you can easily recognize your own Achilles' heel.

YOUR AFTER-FIVE HOURS
NEED A REAL UPPER,
NOT AN ARTIFICIAL DOWNER

I'm convinced that for most adult Americans the standard twilight exercise, the evening's drink or drinks, is a response to their recognition that they must do something to untense. You know as well as I the many reasons why alcohol is essentially bad for people. But let me provide you with one more (which I hope will lead you to a momentous, life-extending decision to first limit your alcoholic intake to wine—and eventually to give it up altogether). The problem with alcohol is that it relaxes you entirely too well, and is a depressant. You have two drinks, deactivate yourself, and manage to retain barely enough spark to sink into a comfortable armchair with a magazine or in front of the television.

Here is the result: To the degree and with the rapidity that your blood sugar zooms, within an hour or so (depending on your movement pattern and evening meal) there will be an equivalent *drop*.

What do you do, then, for a pickup at the end of your day's work? Before you leave your place of business, or a half-hour before dinner, nibble on a healthful blood-sugar builder: a cup of hot broth and just a small piece of cheese eaten slowly; or a few raisins and sunflower seeds and a small apple. Within thirty or forty minutes, when your body has had time to react to these energy-boosters, you will feel a surge of energy. Advise yourself this is going to happen and be ready to notice that zinger of vitality when it strikes.

FOR AN ALL-OVER
PATTERN, MIX AND MATCH

Mix and match elements from the basic approaches. You may wish to add two minutes of rope-jumping to your showering and makeup time in the morning; *and* walk to the market every day; *and* reserve half an hour before dinner to put a twilight twinkle into your eye. Fine, so long as you remember to include at least one real segment of sustained exertion somewhere in your daily plan.

Draw up a list of
1. Different kinds of exercises and sports
2. Exercise classes available where you live
3. Physical chores you perform around your home

Rate them by dividing them into three categories: the ones you like very, very much; those you can tolerate; and what you cannot stand. Select accordingly. It's your plan, intended to last you a lifetime, so let it reflect your personality and style. Improvise. Observe your own reactions (may they be joyous).

In time, like a Washington, D.C., journalist I know, you may make up your own rules. She gave a dinner in my honor on one of my regular autumn trips to the East, and I couldn't refrain from remarking how slim and marvelous she looked. She had undergone a becoming weight change since we first met. Her husband raised his glass to both of us. "To Deborah," he said. "You've changed my life. Among other things, I know that it's morning when my wife is wearing her blue jogging suit, and that it's bedtime when she's in her red leotard. The only difference between our house and Stillman's Gym is that our place smells better."

RED LEOTARD IN THE BLUE OF THE NIGHT?

Red leotard at bedtime? I must have looked puzzled. "I'm on the evening pattern," my reporter friend explained, "but with one twist—I do half an hour of spot exercises just before going to bed.

"I know you say they should be done to music but since we have no record player upstairs in our bedroom I watch television to amuse myself. It doesn't get me too pepped up to go to bed, as it does some people. I'll sit down for ten minutes or so afterward, then go straight to bed, and I'm ready for sleep."

The early-morning part of her day's activity consists

of a mile-and-a-quarter jog before breakfast. It takes her about twelve minutes. (At the time of her first visit to the Golden Door three years before, she had never jogged; as of last year, her husband joins her and runs three miles a day.)

I walk a great many places I never would have before. I hop a cab only when it's too far to go and I don't have time to walk it. And after my last trip to the Golden Door I skied better and longer than I ever dreamed possible. I just have a lot more stamina, a lot more fun now because of the constant exercise—and because I'm thinner.

UPSTAIRS, DOWNSTAIRS

Another guest tells me that what she does at the office and elsewhere is to walk up and down stairs wherever she can find them. In an elevator culture, that occasionally arouses some peculiar looks. The last time she was in Chicago, staying on the eighth floor of a hotel, she found the stairs after much searching and started walking up and down them. The hotel maintenance people who used the stairs began to recognize her. One day, as she passed the third floor, one of the men opened the door for her, thinking she was a run-of-the-mill guest going from one floor to another. Then he took a second look and said, "Oh, that's right, you're *that* one!"

I would guess that anticipation makes exercising twice the work: once when you think about it and again when you do it. Don't think about it. Do it.

INSPIRE THE CHILD WITHIN

FIND FELICITOUS, IMAGINATIVE SURROUNDINGS. You choose to dine in pretty restaurants rather than eating in dull and dreary surroundings. Why not similarly stage-design your physical activity?

Do you have a nearby park with greenery and knolls and winding paths and a soft springy turf? Use it. Explore all of it. Why jog around only the edge, next to the exhaust fumes? To have fresh air, sunshine, and living grass and trees around us is always a treat for the senses under any circumstances.

Do you have a garden of your own? Use it as a background for exercising. You can use the natural perfume of all outdoors to reactivate your breathing apparatus. If you're a city dweller and you're generally confined indoors, the plant shop on your block can help you bring the world of nature into your apartment.

When exercising indoors choose your largest room, preferably one with large windows, and open them all the way. If furniture is cramping you, move it aside. You want space in which to breathe deeply and to kick out all the kinks.

USE MUSIC TO ORCHESTRATE YOUR EXERCISES. Music creates good feeling and keeps movement flowing naturally. At first, just put on your favorite music as background. Later you can start moving in tempo with the beat. The advantage, beyond the sheer euphony of it all, is that music can cue you to what exercise movement comes next.

If you don't know any hard-driving or amusing get-up-and-get-with-it music, let me tell you about *Chicken Fat,* the contagious, fast-moving exercise record so well liked it's sold a half-million a year ever since it was suggested by the Kennedy administration's emphasis on physical fitness. As a public service, the U.S. Junior Chamber of Commerce, Post Office Box 7, Tulsa, Oklahoma 74103, will send you a *Chicken Fat* record, at cost, for only $1.00. Besides the name, mention its catalog number, 865-8. It's 60¢ when ordered in quantities of twenty-five or more.

REWARD YOURSELF. Chances are you don't receive nearly as much physical attention as you did when you were six years old—yet the child within you still adores it. You can harness that feeling to motivate yourself, in the same way that the Golden Door helps guests persevere in some very tough routines. We supply various "strokes" as lavish reward for hard work. Arranged around Japanese gardens and courtyards are salons replete with facials and therapeutic Swedish massages and herbal wraps.

One distinguished psychoanalyst told me he was outraged by these "decadent frills"—that is, until the end of his first day when, as he sank with relief onto the massage table, he realized how richly he deserved to be stroked and catered to like a king. He had earned it.

REWARD YOURSELF. Your rewards to yourself needn't be elaborate. If you can afford to install a sauna, a steam cabinet, or a Japanese hot tub, don't hesitate. Any of these will beautifully soothe your hardworking body. But just an occasional facial or beauty treatment can make you feel as if you've been decorated with honors.

Not all the payoffs need be physically therapeutic. A ticket to a concert, an afternoon off for window-shopping, or a long-postponed tea with some friends are other ways of telling your psyche, "Congratulations!"

SHARE WORKOUTS WITH FRIENDS, OLD AND NEW. Doing anything with a friend intensifies the experience, so enroll together in a class in dance-exercise, or form one. Your initial aches and eventual triumphs should be shared with others who are like-minded. A special sort of fellowship often develops among such classmates, and you may find your life expanding with new friends as you wonder how you ever managed without them. You can swap exercise ideas, lighten occasional moments of gloom—and applaud each other's progress.

This spring the Detroit *News* saluted several local ladies who have set up gyms in their own homes. Pretty Lynn Davidson, wife of an auto-industry executive, likes to exercise with friends. She has plenty of takers for her invitations to work out in a gym described as "half the size of a basketball court." A session was in progress there when the *News* reporter recorded how Lynn has reproduced her version of the Golden Door:

HOW MO-TOWN MOVES
INTO HIGH GEAR

Along with a half-dozen friends who arrive in leotards and tights right after they have sent their children to school, Mrs. Davidson exercises for 90 minutes three or four times a week.

They loosen up by grabbing basketballs and shooting several baskets.

Then Mrs. Davidson takes over, putting on an exercise tape recording made for her when she was a visitor at the Golden Door. . . .

Arms stretch, bodies bend and twist, waistlines writhe, legs flail in all directions as Mrs. Davidson calls out the exercises. . . .

Thirty minutes into the calisthenics, she calls for a fruit break. The friends adjourn to a kitchen-lounge adjoining the gym to devour a tray of juicy orange slices.

One woman picks up a cigarette, and the others register their dismay. She snuffs it out quickly and settles for a few bites of the fruit.

"Back to work," says the reed-slim Mrs. Davidson, and her troops obey. Spreading towels on the floor, they launch into a series of intricate leg exercises, designed to whittle thighs and buttocks.

They are followed by a new tape featuring balletic movements. Hardly the powder-puff type, they are demanding and require a considerable amount of dancing skill.

Another break is called, this one for ice cubes. "It's how they do it at the Golden Door," explains Mrs. Davidson. . . .

The class winds up with the friends skipping rope around the gym.

Next August Mrs. Davidson and a friend . . . are planning to open a men's shop featuring European fashions. . . .

"Somehow I'll work the exercising in along with the business."

IMAGERY AND EXERCISES

Your body finds joy in a spectrum of movement.

Let imagination lift you: Focus on the sensations within your body whenever you exercise. You are going to appreciate them more and more. Since the act of seeing distracts your attention from your body, from time to time close your eyes as you move. Occasionally you may wish to go through some movements in slow motion, concentrating on the muscles that control the movement, and relaxing others.

Try these six visualizations:

1. FEEL THE FORCE OF GRAVITY. The most efficient and graceful movement occurs when your muscles and bones are perfectly aligned with gravity as they go about their work. Another word for this is *balance*. Feel for balance as you move. Flex forward and back and sideways as you exercise, until you reach that central point of balance where all your forces are aligned with gravity and none is being dissipated in the strain of misalignment.

2. MOVE FROM YOUR CENTER. The big muscle masses that should take care of your heavy work are located close to the vertical axis of the body, the spine. When you stand sideways to the mirror, ideally you want your ears, the tips of your shoulders, your hip-bones, and your anklebones to line up. You win a bonus in balance when they do, as well as an easy elegant posture that is admired for itself alone.

Imagine that every movement of your arms and legs is initiated by the spine. You'll discover that you now are in *perfect* balance, using muscles close to your core.

Here's an amazing footnote to the importance of good posture at all times. It comes from Kavner and Dusky, and their book *Total Vision*. They say postural imbalance can so affect all body processes that it may even distort your vision.

3. MOVE LENGTHWISE. All muscles have to contract to do their work, but some tend to remain contracted even when not working. These produce extra tension

which the working muscles have to fight against, reducing the body's efficiency.

Many people don't even know that the muscles of the neck near the shoulders are usually contracted and tense. As you run or work out, imagine a string is attached to the top of your head, pulling upward and gently stretching your spine, elongating your body. Drop your shoulders. Focus on your spine and loosen all the muscle groups that are binding it, shortening it, and stiffening it. Soon you'll feel a stretching, lengthening effect that is also a new relaxation.

4. MOVE ABOUT ON ALL FOURS. Have a favorite animal? Imagine yourself as that animal. Move around as it does and imitate its characteristic rhythm. You will use many an unaccustomed muscle. Of itself, crawling is a great restorer of body balance because it makes you so very aware of your spine.

5. MOVE BACK INTO TIME. Play primitive or ethnic music; or music of some specific time and place. I love the English morris dances ("Greensleeves" is the best-known example). Fantasize the music. Live it.

6. MOVE LIGHTLY. Here's another example of the interaction of mind and body. Point your elbows down and hold them firmly in position as a friend puts her hands under them and tries to lift you off the ground. You can make yourself seem lighter to her by visualizing yourself as weightless, as part of a current of energy pouring up and through you toward the sky. But if you picture yourself as inert, she'll have a great deal more trouble lifting you.

Obviously, you always can make your movement seem light and buoyant by picturing yourself that way. This is just another facet, just another quality of excellence, of vitality, that exercise can add to your life.

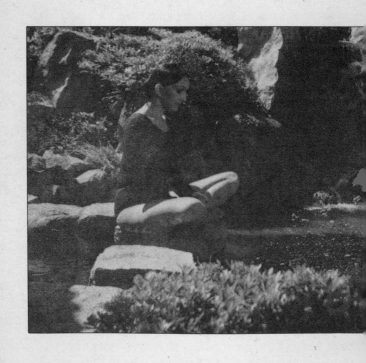

CHAPTER III

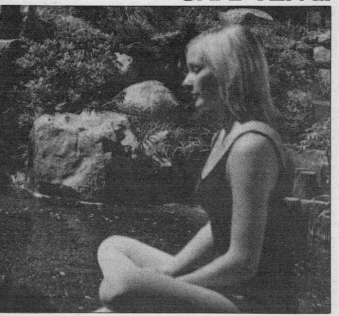

BODY
AWARENESS:
ANOTHER SOURCE
OF BEAUTY

Thence is a saying that all brides are beautiful, and it's true, because for a little while, the young woman being married has everyone's permission to focus all her attention on herself. I have never seen a bride approach an altar with bad posture. It is this ability to be aware of herself that separates an attractive woman from a plain one.

You can keep your own excitement alive even though you are not a bride. Listen to your senses. That is the first step in this exciting journey that you and I have set out upon. You have a whole new world to explore, full of unknown resources and inspirations. It starts at your skin and proceeds inward.

Your body wants to feel healthy. Your muscles are eager to move. If you will open up your senses to learn what your body is trying to tell you, you will find it your most reliable guide. The fact is, true health and beauty come from no external source; they come from within yourself. When you look into the new world under your skin, you will find that exploring it will be the greatest adventure you have ever known.

YOUR 1980s GLAMOUR: LEADING FROM TENSILE (NOT TINSEL) STRENGTH

Your only guide should be what makes you feel good. You have already made a big move in the direction of feeling fine by choosing the first essential of well-being—regular physical activity. But don't rely on sheer willpower alone to make your exercise last a lifetime. There are two marvelous additional essentials available to you—relaxation and joy.

Instead of drifting thoughtlessly through your physical activities, become newly aware of your body as you let your movements be guided and personalized by your senses. Make contact with the flow of feelings that

1. ensures that your daily activities are adapted to the needs of your life and your body;

2. helps you to banish tension and feel the full benefits of exercise;

3. opens a whole new realm of delightful sensations that expand, enrich, and sustain your health and beauty program.

Soon you will notice that you have plenty of company, because, as you experience your senses and your body awakens, as your skin begins to glow and your eyes to sparkle, others around you will share the same excitement. In some mysterious way, people who delight in themselves delight others as well.

EXPERIENCING YOUR BODY

In recent years there has been an explosion of information about food, exercise, and health in general.

How do you judge what is valid? How can you choose what is healthy for you?

Amid all the conflicting advice, there is one way, and one alone, for you to know what is good for you. Listen to your body. Pay attention to what your senses are telling you. Awareness of breathing, muscle tension, skin sensations, heartbeat—these and other interior processes, as well as good elimination, sound sleep, and hearty appetite, are your key checkpoints.

It is not difficult. I'm not asking you to achieve the kind of total control over the body that a yogi has. What I want you to do is to get to know yourself and to bring balance into your sensory world by listening to what your body is telling you. For years, your messages have come from "out there"; now you are going to spend some time listening to "in here."

Have you been a puritan up to now? Have you been one of those people who are afraid that too much sensuality will distract them from higher intellectual or spiritual pursuits, who insist that there are more important things in life than pampering the body? Believe me, a healthy body, over whose workings you have control, will never hinder you from striving for these higher goals. Indeed, a sound body is the greatest aid to freeing your mind. It puts you in control and lets you make the choices.

HOW A WRITER
LEARNED BODY
READ-OUT

Making contact with a long-dormant body presents some people with forms of excitement they hadn't counted on. Blair Sabol, one of the busiest writers in America, who often writes on fashion and beauty, used to pay some attention to her body, mostly by doing stretches and bends whenever she thought of it. After her first visit to the Golden Door, she found herself paying more attention to aerobics and to the feedback her body gives her, so she takes a morning walk on the beach when she can—"but there are times when that's hard for me, especially if I stay out past twelve o'clock the night before."

"What I do manage to do," she said, "every single day in Los Angeles, is to take an exercise class." She went on:

> . . . an hour and a half of huffy-puffy work. I have the kind of body that has to move a lot before I feel anything, so this class is like a bunch of Body Awakeners all in a row.
>
> It's a damned nuisance, to be frank. I have to take it early in the morning or late in the evening so I can construct a day around it. But it's my therapy. A lot of my friends are going to shrinks, and I'm putting the time and money toward getting to know my body. Maybe I'm getting as much as they are; we'll see.

HOW TO OPERATE
WITH OPERANT CONDITIONING

She barely paused for breath before the rush of words continued.

> I did find one thing about the Door that was disconcerting. You know, by the middle of the week I found myself doing all the movement, eating the food with gusto, feeling absolutely terrific about myself. My body got revved up—and then, a week or two after I left the Door, something happened—a big mental drop.
>
> I had just experienced myself being in the best shape I'd ever been in, as if every muscle was cleaned and toned and sparkling, and for once I knew what it must feel like to be an athlete.

Blair decided that the problem lay in going home to the old stimuli that made old habits want to come back. She sees her walk and the exercise class as ways to hold on to the Golden Door experience.

Awareness of the way her body feels, however,

comes to Blair's rescue even when it isn't entirely comfortable.

I figured out that I can do a lot of little things as triggers for my Door experience every day out here in the real world. That's why I try to do something every day that reminds me of the Door. The walk, the exercise class, tricks with food. If I miss two days in a row of that exercise class, I start feeling the slippage. . . . I am plagued with the fear that I'm addicted to the Door.

YOUR MESSENGERS: THE SENSES

All your knowledge about the world and about your body comes to you, of course, through your sensory systems, so let's examine them briefly. As you read and experience these sensations, contemplate the miracles that lie within your body; it is as much an energy center as is the universe, and it is yours to direct.

We all have not just the traditional five senses of sight, hearing, taste, smell, and touch. We actually have seven. The extra two are kinesthesia (the sense of position and movement in the body) and balance (provided by the inner ear).

I call kinesthesia and balance, along with touch from among the traditional five senses, the "body" senses, since they provide you with information about what is going on inside your body. Just because they aren't "head" senses like the first four—that is, they aren't used primarily to provide information about what is happening out in the world—you must not forget to cultivate them.

Take a look at the two extra senses, kinesthesia and balance.

KINESTHESIA. This real sixth sense is at least as complex and mysterious as ESP, the supposed "sixth sense" that some researchers are convinced we can develop. For a simple demonstration of kinesthesia, close your eyes and touch your nose with a fingertip.

Now think: How do you know that your finger is moving toward your nose?

You have millions of nerve endings with specialized sense organs built into all the muscle tissue of your body. As each muscle tenses and relaxes, complex messages are transmitted to your brain, which "charts" the progress of the movement being made.

There are not only nerve hookups to the voluntary skeletal muscles; we also receive information from the heart, from the muscles that push our food through the intestines, and from other muscles which do all the other routine work of the body. The result is that we have the potential for knowing what is happening anywhere within our bodies at any given moment. The same nervous system tells us how much strain each muscle is undergoing.

The formal word for the nerve endings that give you such important bodily information is interoceptors.

BALANCE. Besides these interoceptors, our bodies have a remarkable organ that lets us know how we are placed and in what direction we are going relative to the ground. It is, of course, the inner ear that provides us with a sense of balance and orientation.

SENSE-STRETCHING. Because all seven senses are at your command, your body is a marvelously flexible device. Remember, your body was designed to be used in a broad array of ways. You need not restrict yourself to a narrow range of movement and sensation.

If you are feeling stale, your problem is not one of sloth. I do not believe that you are lazy, and that you indolently lie around the house all day doing nothing. But you might be leading a "steady-state" life: that is, you might be moving through the same repetitive daily activities, almost as though you had been programmed, so that the muscles and the senses you haven't been using are sluggish.

We have learned at the Golden Door to alternate between vigorous exercise and voluptuous relaxation, not just to give hardworking bodies a rest but also to open up the whole thrilling range of awareness that is available to everyone. Just as some movements are designed to awaken your muscles, so relaxation allows your senses to move into new, undiscovered freedom.

Discover for yourself your own repertoire of sense-stretchers. A good way to start is to give yourself a chance to exercise your awareness as consciously as you exercise your muscles. If you can take a whole day off, fine. If not, make a quiet place within your day, an hour or two if you can. But remember, you are setting aside this time for you to do things for yourself, not for others. Ignore any charges of vanity or selfishness as you find ways and make the time to do these awareness exercises.

SIGHT. Strive for a broad range of visual input, long-range and close-up, quick-scanning and point-watching. Caress a variety of visual textures with your eyes. Trace crisp outlines and bright colors in strong sunshine; in duskiness, soften your focus and pay attention to the masses and backgrounds of your visual field. At night, turn out some of the lights in your living room to create some contrast between areas of darkness and pools of brightness.

Here are four specific exercises to relax and freshen the eyes. Repeat each one as often as you can without discomfort.

1. *Eye Painting*. Stand relaxed with your arms hanging loosely. Begin swinging your body from side to side. When you feel secure, close your eyes for a few seconds, then open them partly so that the world is just a blur passing by. Finally open your eyes completely, without focusing. Swing your eyes right to left, then left to right. Imagine your sweep of vision as a paintbrush making horizontal strokes. Just enjoy the shapes and color impressions flashing by, without trying to give them meaning or outline.

2. *Range-Switching*. If you are reading or doing other close work, periodically look up and out at some distant object, giving your eyes a break by changing the focal length of the lens. Switch back and forth from close up to far away.

3. *Blinking*. It breaks the strain of looking steadily. Simply blink in a slow, regular rhythm, concentrating

on the muscles around the eyes, relaxing them, getting rid of squinting and other tensions. Vary the speed next, moving to a rapid flutter.

4. *Eyeball Rolling.* Rotate your eyes in their sockets, not too hard. Go clockwise, then counterclockwise, trying to catch the shadows that are made at the peripheries by your eyelids.

HEARING. Aim for the same kind of contrast you gave your eyes. Focus on the smaller sounds that are normally drowned in the blast of traffic and household noise: crickets, the closing of a window, or the soft susurrus of a breeze in the trees.

TASTE. We need never worry about the tongue muscle being under-exercised. Seldom is it idle. It works hard to help us speak and is even more industrious at mealtime. The tongue performs a muscular marathon, pushing food back beyond the teeth, mixing food with saliva, then helping push the food back for swallowing (a function which it performs even when we humans are in the fetal state). See also "Glorious Eating" (page 241) and the recipes at the back of the book.

A noted authority on taste and smell urges variety in everything when dinner is served. And he would have you revel in all your senses in order to sharpen your appreciation of food. For visual effect, he recommends frequent changes of table decorations and dishes (a daily practice at the Golden Door, where each meal is an individual feast for the eye, on dishes that make it a *trompe l'oeil* as well).

Because your gratified, preoccupied senses will be staggering under this sensory onslaught, small servings will be sure to suffice.

SMELL. Seek out the less strident odors. Perfume your sheets so that when you go to bed you can imagine yourself submerged in deep, soft fragrance. Place scents in handbags, dress linings, anywhere that will give pleasure to you and those around you. Surround yourself with flowers, a few growing plants, and a touch of incense now and then. Be aware of the dry scent of rocks baking under the sun, of newly mowed lawns, of baking bread, of fresh new breezes—there are hundreds of lovely smells we take for granted.

Touch? Remember those standbys, the hot dinner plate and the chilled salad dish—and the simple thrill of the chilled salad fork. Sound? On special occasions, present the spitting sizzle of a spinach salad flambé, with all its attendant theatrics. The expert suggests you learn to take pleasure in less obvious sounds, too, as for example the bubbling of Perrier water.

You probably know that the skin is a single, complex organ—the largest of all our organs. Forming the physical boundary of our selves, it contains one of the most basic sensory systems, the sense of touch. Touch has been called the "mother of senses" because it develops in the embryo earlier than any other sense.

Notice that when you really want to verify the existence of something, you want to touch it. Lovers are always touching each other. Touching, in short, is one of the basic ways to communicate emotion, and we all need our quota of caresses, given and received.

On a less emotional level, you can greatly increase your awareness of the sheer information that comes to you through your skin. A few of the areas are:

Texture. Think how much poorer your life would be if you could never distinguish the difference in texture between moss, grasses, a handful of rich loam, or autumn leaves. Try sleeping nude and be conscious of the sleek sheets and their cool folds against your body.

Pressure. Have you ever played the game in which someone writes on your back with a finger while you try to decipher the message? The skin is amazingly sensitive to variations in pressure. When you step from your bath, play afterbath pat-a-cake, giving yourself gentle pats all over at a moderately brisk tempo, just before toweling off. Pat with one finger, with a flat hand, with cupped hands, and use varying degrees of force. After a little such conditioning, you'll react to even the subtlest distinctions in pressure.

Temperature and Humidity. The touch of the air upon the skin when you step outdoors tells you whether the atmosphere is balmy or frigid, muggy or arid. The next time you reach into the oven, notice that just for an instant you can detect the boundary between the hot air inside and the cold air outside. Vary the temperature of your shower: from warm to hot, to very hot, to cool, to icy cold.

YOUR POSTURE: A GAUGE OF KINESTHESIA AND BALANCE

To remind yourself of the precision with which you can enjoy kinesthesia and balance, go back to the chapter on movement and run through the six visualizations of feeling the force of gravity, moving from your center, moving lengthwise, moving lightly, and moving to music. As you practice each one, observe how you hold yourself during the exercise and also later while sitting, standing, resting, and performing everyday routines. It's your body alignment that you're regarding now with a critical eye.

The next time you watch your body move, have in mind these little secrets of proper alignment:

1. As you stand tall, squeeze your buttock muscles tautly.

2. While walking, pretend you're carrying a jug of water in the graceful Balinese manner. With one steadying hand hold the jug aloft on your shoulder or high on your head. You will feel so tall and lithe.

3. Pretend you're a night-running locomotive. There's a powerful light shining from the center of your chest, boring through the blackness. Your job is to keep the beam aimed straight at the track ahead.

PSST! IT'S YOUR POSTURE

Your posture continually sends messages in two directions. Inwardly, it reports the ways your body responds to gravity, to the muscular demands of any task you set yourself, and to your state of mind. All of this influences your vitality. Distorted posture means your muscles can't work efficiently, and your energy is being sapped as muscle groups struggle against one another instead of cooperating.

Outwardly, posture is your body's statement about how vital and attractive and strong you feel. If you permit your stomach muscles to go too slack, your spine will curve and a "pot" will protrude in front. Shoulders also will slope forward to compensate, the chin will drop, and wrinkles and double chins will form. Your carriage always is sending a distinct message about you to the world outside.

I grew up with dreadful posture—a tendency to hunch my head forward. I'm convinced it was because of an attitude toward life I developed when I was very young. Today I have improved my posture sufficiently not to mind talking about it.

As the first child I took on a good deal of responsibility very early in life. My mother refused to take care of household finances; my father would give me a check and, from the time I was thirteen, I budgeted for us all. Then came marriage at seventeen and the responsibility of running Rancho La Puerta and handling dozens of staff people, some of them two or three times my age. It all added up to my feeling that the world was sitting on my back. I became more and more hunched.

ABOUT THE RABBIT
AND THE TURTLE—IT'S NO FABLE

Someone more timid than I might have pushed her nose ahead of her like a rabbit; another, more defensive, might have pulled her head in like a turtle. It's hard to be outgoing and expansive if you have the stance of either a rabbit or a turtle.

The first step in changing ourselves is often a matter of changing our posture. If you can stand tall and loose, head up and feet well planted, you feel—and look—like a person centered between the earth and the skies. Good posture is particularly important as one grows older because bad posture inhibits breathing. You need the full capacity of your lungs to supply oxygen to your

---

brain. So sit and stand tall. This will directly affect your behavior and the response of everyone you meet.

Through kinesthesia and balance there are several ways to build a simple, erect, and efficient stance. Try these:

1. THE MARIONETTE. I like the image of a strong, invisible silken cord pulling me up from the solar plexus, through to the center of my head, as if I were a puppet on a string. To imagine the tug of the cord, the stretch, the upward trend, will make me elongate my body line every time I think of it.

2. YOUR DIAPHRAGM AS A CONCERTINA. I always remember to stand tall when I think of my diaphragm as a concertina I can expand and stretch wa-a-ay out, just as an accordionist does when he performs.

3. BONESTACKING. Your bones are designed to carry the weight of your body; your muscles, to move it. But when the skeleton's alignment is all out of kilter, the muscles have to do support duty as well and you're going to feel tired in a hurry.

In your mind, try to picture each bone. Tell yourself to feel how each portion of the bone structure rests solidly on the one below. Be aware of gravity passing vertically through your whole body frame.

4. ELIMINATING VISUAL INPUT. Close your eyes and stand straight, arms held out to the sides at right angles. Lift one knee above your waist and try to hold it there for ten seconds. Equalize the muscle tensions all over your body. Don't let them localize—you'll topple.

Take other positions while you stand with your eyes closed and rely completely on your kinesthetic sense.

5. THE BODY PLEDGE OF ALLEGIANCE. My reflection in a looking-glass or a shop window makes me think of my morning exercise time (and that full-length mirror) and draw myself up. That's why in looking at photographs of myself today and thirty years ago I see such a marked difference in my posture. I now have a posture that proclaims my happiness. People who haven't seen me for many years always say, "You've lost weight!" (I haven't.) Or they exclaim, "You look so much younger!" (Of course I'm not.)

SENSORY UNDERLOAD

You must provide yourself with contrast and change in order to function with all systems at go. But, exactly as too little activity can cause the senses to atrophy, so can too much. You'll simply blank out if you're bombarded too steadily with an overload of stimuli.

For refreshment you need occasional periods of sensory underload. For one day, or even two or three, give your taste buds a rest with the Virtue-Making Diet (page 297). From time to time, sit for half an hour in silence. Turn out the lights at twilight and rest your eyes in the dusty-lilac dusk. Turn off.

Dr. John Lilly, who became celebrated for his research with dolphins, has carried the concept of sensory deprivation to its logical extreme in his experimental work. Inside his "Lilly tank"—a container of salty body-temperature water—a human research subject floats with eyes and ears covered, and nothing at all to touch. Subjects report that, as senses go into eclipse, their inner imagery and other forms of consciousness shoot off on new and sometimes unexpected tangents.

HOW INNER COMMUNICATIONS
ARE SHORT-CIRCUITED

Although the three "body" senses (touch, balance, and kinesthesia) also enable us to know our physical selves in almost infinite detail, most of the information flowing through our skin and interoceptors never gets through to consciousness. Somewhere along the line it is shut out.

For example, how often are you aware of your digestion? Most of us know nothing about what is happening in our intestines unless a gross disorder occurs and a red-flagged message finally gets through.

There are two barriers to perfect communication via the body senses. Luckily, both can be overcome. The first is merely lack of education. Many of us are sensory illiterates who were never taught to be aware of our skin, our motions, and our balance. The remedy lies in simple exercises such as those in this chapter. The second barrier is tension. Many of us have learned to shut off the sometimes painful flow of information from the body. We do this by muscle-clenching. This powerful inhibitor of our body senses is the state doctors call stress and most of us call tension.

THE DIS-EASE OF TENSION

After years of considering my problems and those of my guests, together we have learned that treating the symptoms of stress is nowhere near as effective as finding ways to develop ease and adroitness in the ways you handle stress. If you're a high achiever with an exciting life, you live with stress. There has to be some of it in every life, but you definitely can learn how to convert tension to creative action.

Tension is basically a physiological reaction to emotion. Whenever a person entertains fear or rage, the body prepares itself for action. Blood pressure rises, pulse and heartbeat quicken, body temperature goes up, digestion slows down, adrenaline pours into the bloodstream. More sugar is then manufactured to feed energy to the muscles. The muscles themselves tighten—and there you have tension buildup.

IDENTIFYING TENSION

Virtually everyone has his or her own body signature —a personal pattern of tension that produces an individual posture and gait.

Try this experiment: Lie down on the floor, on your back, and relax. If you are truly relaxed, almost all of your spine will touch the floor except for a few vertebrae in the small of your back. If you have tension in the lower back, a common place for it, your spine will arch away from the floor.

Now, while you are still relaxed and on your back, your arms lying slack with the palms down, raise the fingers of your left hand as high as you can. Just bend your wrist back, nothing else. Focus your attention on the upper forearm and the muscle there that you clenched to bend your wrist. Feel the muscle with your mind; that is the sensation of tension. Get to know it, so you can recognize it elsewhere in your body.

Some other very common centers of tension are:

1. Forehead and scalp: Tense muscles here are major contributors to headaches and eye aches.

2. Jaw: Tooth-grinding and clenching of the jaw can cause pain.

3. Nape of neck: Another contributor to headaches, fatigue, and general feelings of rigidity.

4. Shoulders: A great fatigue-producer; tension here easily spreads to the neck and produces a headache.

5. Stomach and abdomen: Tension here is often associated with ulcers (although it does not cause them directly).

6. Buttocks and anus: Colon disorders are a possible result of chronic tension here.

No matter where the tension is, you will know it by its pain—a headache, a dull muscle ache that is quite different from the twinge you might feel in a muscle you just used for the first time in months—and by the most reliable indicator, fatigue. You know the fatigue I mean —not the pleasant tiredness of an exercised body, but the draggy feeling you wake up with after what should have been a good night's sleep.

EXERCISES TO DISSOLVE TENSION

Return to your position on the floor, on your back. Strain your left wrist backward just as you did before. Let your hand fall back to the floor, of its own weight. Now feel the forearm, in your mind. Don't make an effort to relax. Real relaxation is neither trying nor doing; rather, it's doing nothing. The forearm muscle feels very different now, doesn't it? Can you sense the increased flow of blood and easy energy? That's the sensation of relaxation.

You can apply the same principle to every muscle

group in your body. For gradual relaxation, you add one extra series of steps: Instead of progressing from full tension to full relaxation in just one jump, do it in stages. Start with that same left arm. Tense it slightly, then a little more and a little more, until after ten seconds the arm has reached maximum rigidity. Now relax in the same small stages, back down to your original limp state. And then concentrate on relaxing your arm even further. Keep on letting go.

If you progressively relax all your muscles in this way, you'll soon be adept at recognizing residual tension and releasing it. Monitor the different muscle groups. Grow familiar with the areas most vulnerable to stress. At various times throughout the day, check to be sure you're not tightening up.

There's another way to vary tension systematically. If you discover a section of your body tensed, try shaking it loose. First the hands and arms, then shoulders and head, feet and legs; finally shimmy the entire body. Now relax and feel that tingle.

THE INS AND OUTS OF
BREATHING FOR RELAXATION

Muscular contraction is just one of the hints your body gives you about tension buildup. Another is shallow, inhibited breathing. The flow of feeling parallels the flow of breath. If you doubt that, notice how you breathe the next time you're confronted by danger or a need for quick action: Your breath crowds into the top half of your chest as part of the fight-or-flight mechanism.

It's impossible to experience your body totally when you're breathing in shallow little gasps. But when you breathe fully and deeply, the body acknowledges a signal that all is safe. Tension drains off, and sensations and feelings flow freely.

That's why almost every mental and physical discipline begins with exercises in breath control. The ancient Hindus revered breath as so precious that they spoke of the measure of human life not in terms of years, but in breaths. Breath control is a profound technique of experiencing and ultimately controlling the dual physical-mental Self.

How do you breathe?

HOW DO *YOU* BREATHE?

Lie with your back flat on the floor. Lift your head slightly as you raise your knees; or, to be completely comfortable, slip a pillow beneath your head. Just breathe normally. Observe. Which parts move with your breathing? Upper chest? Stomach? Back? Does one side breathe more pronouncedly than the other? Does your neck tense as you breathe in?

Sense your abdomen and diaphragm, the latter being the large muscle separating your inner chest from your inner abdomen. The diaphragm is the workhorse of the respiratory system. It contracts and plunges down toward the stomach, creating a hollow into which air rushes. This pushes the abdominal organs down toward the pelvis, and slightly outward, so the stomach and lower back swell a little. Exhalation is a passive process: The diaphragm just lets go, relaxes to its original position, shoving the lungs back up until they have no room for all that air. As the air is expelled, the rib cage shrinks, along with the volume of the lungs.

Tension in the rib cage, back, or stomach muscles can keep the lungs from expanding to their fullest. Try some tests: As the diaphragm contracts downward, feel your lower back. Make sure those muscles and ribs are free to expand. This back breathing is very important. It means the air is rushing to the very bottom of the lungs. Now do the same with your side ribs. Are they as loose as they should be? Do they expand laterally as you inhale? Move your hands to your chest and feel it rise with each inhalation. Make sure there's no constriction in your chest. Finally, put your fingers to your collarbones, to determine whether breath is entering all the way to the top of the thorax. Do your collarbones rise as you breathe in?

A SIMPLE INTRODUCTION
TO YOGA BREATHING

Having checked yourself over, you're ready to do two favorite yoga breathing exercises, Ha Breathing and The Lion:

1. HA BREATHING. Stand with your arms at your sides. Your feet should be at least a shoulder's width apart. The palms of your hands are turned inward.

First breathe out, voiding your lungs *completely.* Then inhale slowly through the nostrils as you lift your arms above your head. Let the upper part of your body fall forward from the hips. As you do so, you needn't utter a sound but you must mouth the word "Ha!" as though you were shouting it while simultaneously exhaling through your mouth.

Let your head and arms dangle. Be sure your neck muscles are equally relaxed. As you straighten up, lift your arms once more above your head as you slowly inhale through your nose. Then drop your arms slowly to your sides, exhaling very slowly, and return to starting position. In the beginning, repeat at least three times; gradually increase to ten times.

2. THE LION. Sit on your heels. Place your palms on your knees. Take a deep breath. Then exhale violently, stretching your jaw down in an exaggerated way and poking out your tongue as far as you can. At the same time, spread your fingers fanwise and stiffen your hands, forming claws. Freeze for a few seconds. Then relax. Repeat at least three times.

Into your exercise program and into every activity of the day, incorporate your newfound awareness of the flow of breath. Delight in its rhythm and tranquillity.

USING TENSION
AS A GROWTH TOOL

It's time to insert a reminder that stress is natural enough and that tension can be useful. Your health and beauty depend upon how well you cope with and master tension. Everything we've cited and discussed so far assures us that the best antidote for nervous tension is to become physically tired.

Golden Door guest Georgiana Sheldon would like to see employers across the country set up exercise rooms where employees could work out muscular kinks and tensions.

"In my opinion, employees would feel better, work better, and enjoy their jobs more," says this vice-chairman of the Civil Service Commission. And she practices what she preaches. Even during the harrowing weeks following the Guatemalan earthquake of February 1976, when Georgiana kept office hours from six A.M. till midnight or past, being in charge of disaster relief for the State Department, she found the time for a few minutes of yoga.

Listen to another woman who uses all her senses and all her energy on the job every day. On a recent trip to New York I stopped by the Condé Nast offices to see art director Rochelle Udell. And I kept thinking of the change in her since her first day at the Golden Door seven months before.

"Well, you know I went to the Golden Door at a time when I really needed it," she recalled.

> I'd been working quite hard. I'd been through a divorce. In a year I'd put on fifty pounds. Except for my work, everything I'd been doing was self-destructive. I couldn't see myself; I literally had padded my life with activities, and with fat, so that there wasn't any center anymore. I didn't know where I was in the middle of all that, and I didn't want to know.

RUNNING TOWARD LIFE

She had been starved for time to be alone with herself. "In two weeks at the Golden Door," she continued,

> I had to come to terms with a number of things, including how to handle the high-pressure kind of

work. We're constantly meeting deadlines against incredible odds . . .

The most efficacious tranquilizer for Rochelle turned out to be running. At first the lesson of the morning walk at the Door helped. Now, after her third visit to the Golden Door, she not only walks to work (a one-mile distance), but begins each day with a run.

> The running established a balance in my life (Energy begets Energy). I now have worked up to a minimum daily run of three miles (and a six- or eight-mile run three times a week), and every tenth day or so I don't run—my body lets me know when to stop. You learn to listen to it. That's the greatest lesson learned at the Door: "Reading one's own body."

> I have mirrored walls in my apartment and am not afraid to look. Deborah, you taught us to begin each day with a "look and see," and insisted that I redo my kitchen so that it is visually satisfying and the gratification need not come entirely from food.

> But the big breakthrough was understanding that I hated regimented exercise classes and I loved sports. I now approach exercise as a way of life, running daily (and playing tennis for fun), and I reward myself with a massage once a week.

MASSAGE AS A REWARD

Touching is such a basic form of communication that it can do all sorts of things to untwist the emotions. Rubbing yourself down with a towel, giving yourself pats and strokes, can make all your skin's nerve ends say "thank you." But massage—being stroked artistically by an expert—makes you feel better still.

Massage is an ancient art which has been practiced by every culture. An expert can take you beyond relaxation and mere good feeling and provide you with an actual healing experience. The process is all fluidity and grace. Everything happens slowly, rhythmically, and quietly. It literally modifies your breathing. Afterward all is smooth as quiet energy surges through you.

Don't schedule a massage till you really want to take the time to unwind and be a completely passive subject. If you can't relax easily, wait until your exercise program is well under way and you're feeling smug and virtuous. When you know you've earned a special treat, it will be easier to surrender to what many people still consider a sybaritic form of relaxation.

Be a comparison shopper if you have no trusted friend to guide you in choosing a masseuse or a masseur. Select someone of the same sex who is licensed and who doesn't make you nervous. It's best at first to go through a health club or a similar institution with a spotless reputation. And you can call an established school of massage instruction, which probably will refer you to legitimate graduates near you, perhaps even to someone who will come to your home. Massage administered in private, familiar surroundings is even more devastating to the tensions. For this reason our Golden Door guests receive daily Swedish massage in their own rooms.

PROGRESSIVE RELAXATION

Even when very, very tired, do you have difficulty falling asleep? Or do you drop off only to waken within an hour or two?

If you have a tape recorder, you can make your own sleep cassette by repeating the following instructions in your slowest, laziest-sounding voice, against lulling music. But if you have no cassette-player-recorder, just learn this simple progressive-relaxation technique in the daytime—and for daytime use, also—so that you won't have to concentrate very actively at night. When the technique becomes completely automatic, use it as a bedtime wind-down.

SOME PRELIMINARY
UNRAVELING FOR YOUR
RAVELED NERVES

Your bed I trust has a firm mattress. If not, spread a comforter or heavy blanket on the floor. Wear something loose-fitting. Before you lie on your back, go through the steps of Rag Doll, the well-known relaxer. Vertebra by vertebra, incline first your head, neck, shoulders, and then let yourself bend over from the hips, head hanging loosely. Pivot from the trunk of your body, letting your upper torso move to the right (head and arms simply dangle and follow the lead of your torso), then around backward describing as nearly perfect a circle as you can, then to the left side and back to front. Reverse the first step as, vertebra by vertebra, you rise to an erect position. But continue, always very slowly and carefully, to tilt your head backward. Then up again, slowly. You're ready to settle on the floor.

It may ease you to slip a small, soft pillow (an herb pillow would be oh so tranquilizing) beneath your knees as you lie supine on the floor. Legs are together, loosely. Close your eyes, and let your arms fall at your sides. If you think at all, think within your body. Imagine your skeletal frame, your position, the balance and counterbalance of each part, and then let go.

LITTLE BY LITTLE,
TO LYRICAL LIMPNESS

This is what you're to tell your tape cassette:

1. "I am raising my arms and dropping them, parallel above my head. And now I'm stretching from head to toe . . . yawning widely . . . wider. I'm holding the stretch and the yawn—1, 2, 3, 4, 5. Then I can go limp.

2. "I'm placing both hands on top of my head and intertwining my fingers there. My arms lie on the floor. At first I'm looking straight ahead. Then, quickly, I turn my head to the left. Look straight ahead again. Quickly, turn my head to the right. Relax.

3. "I'm letting my chin drop, and all my face is relaxing with it. Just let go, for 1, 2, 3, 4, 5.

4. "I'm slipping my hands behind my neck and locking my fingers. Then I press the back of my head downward against the resistance of my hands. 1, 2, 3, 4, 5. And I go limp.

5. "I put my left thumb in my left armpit; right thumb, right armpit. My upper arms I hold against my sides. Now I'll try to bring my shoulderblades together. 1, 2, 3, 4, 5. Then I'm limp again.

6. "So now I place left hand on left shoulder; right hand, right shoulder. My arms are like little wings lying against the floor. And I flex my biceps for a count: 1, 2, 3, 4, 5. I let my biceps and all relax.

7. "I drop my arms at my sides. I stiffen my elbows. I raise my arms slightly to hold them rigidly while I count: 1, 2, 3, 4, 5. My arms go limp.

8. "Hands, become fists. Now, tense for a count: 1, 2, 3, 4, 5. Go limp at my sides.

9. "I'm trying to bring my shoulders up to my ears. I'm holding tensely for 1, 2, 3, 4, 5. And I relax. Now I'm lifting my shoulders again and also hunching them forward. I'm holding tightly—1, 2, 3, 4, 5. Relax.

10. "I'm frowning so hard that my (creamed) face must be making an awful grimace. And I hold—1, 2, 3, 4, 5. Relax.

11. "I'm lifting my eyebrows high, so high that my scalp feels the pressure from my wrinkled (and well-creamed) forehead. I hold. 1, 2, 3, 4, 5. Relax, eyebrows.

12. "I'm squeezing my eyes (I'm wearing eye cream), till they're very, very tightly shut. Also I'm pouting as hard as I can. I hold tight, 1, 2, 3, 4, 5. Relax, eyes. Unpout, mouth.

13. "Open, eyes. Quickly, I'm peering as far as I can, making my eyes dart left, right, and up, down. Look, look; look, look. Now I'm closing my eyes to place my gently cupped palms over them, shutting out all light. At the same time as I palm my eyes—so soothing—I'm taking five normal breaths and concentrating upon the air entering and leaving my lungs.

14. "My tongue is pressing hard against the roof of my mouth now; 1, 2, 3, 4, 5. Relax. Next, I'm rolling my tongue back, against the roof of my mouth and holding —1, 2, 3, 4, 5. Relax.

15. "My arms are still lying at my sides. I'm clenching my fists again, and at the same time clenching my teeth. 1, 2, 3, 4, 5. Go limp.

16. "I'm pressing my chin to my chest so I can hold for a count. 1, 2, 3, 4, 5. As I relax, I let my head roll quickly to the left. I press my chin to my chest again, and count some more—1, 2, 3, 4, 5. Then I let my head roll to the right. And everywhere I go limp.

17. "I'm fantasizing that my head and shoulders are so terribly heavy. In fact, they're sinking. Tonight, shall it be a warm, shallow pool? Or an obliging fleecy cloud that turns into a large down-filled satin pillow? My head and shoulders are sinking farther and farther, deeper and deeper.

"Now I'm pausing to take several breaths, holding each breath, then exhaling completely. Inhale . . . exhale. Inhale . . . exhale. Inhale . . . exhale. With the exhale, I force the air out of my lungs so that the next intake of air will be greater. . . .

"I'm taking an intermission between my upper body and my lower body.

"I'm placing my arms flat above my head, parallel to each other. I'm imagining that my arms and shoulders are literally pulling away from my body, as if they were moving out with a tide. As I stretch, I'm making more room in my rib cage. I'll inhale once, hold, and exhale slowly. . . .

18. "I'm checking to see that my arms are relaxed and comfortably at my sides again. I'm tensing my stomach muscles. I'm counting once more—1, 2, 3, 4, 5. Go limp.

19. "I'm arching my back for a count—1, 2, 3, 4, 5. I'm letting my spine unroll back down to the floor as I carefully relax.

20. "I'm pressing down with my midriff, with my lower back, carefully. 1, 2, 3, 4, 5. And I relax.

21. "Tense up, buttocks, hard. 1, 2, 3, 4, 5. Relax.

22. "I'm raising my head slightly as I lift my legs about twelve inches from the floor, keeping my knees straight. My left toe points as I stretch my left leg. Hold tightly, left leg. 1, 2, 3, 4, 5. Go limp.

"I'm raising my legs with straight knees again. Point, right toe, and stretch, right leg. 1, 2, 3, 4, 5. Go limp.

23. "In the same position again, with my legs lifted and knees straight, head slightly raised, I tense my thighs. 1, 2, 3, 4, 5. Go limp.

24. "Raising my head and lifting my legs, I'm clasping my hands behind my knees and rolling myself up as if I'm going to kiss my knees. 1, 2, 3, 4, 5. Take it slow and easy, vertebrae, as my spine unrolls back onto floor. Relax. Totally."

YOUR RELAXATION
AFTERGLOW

If you have recorded onto a cassette, time it so that some soporific music still has several minutes' playing time.

Lie fully relaxed for a few minutes, feeling heavy, heavy, heavy, as if the surface you're resting on is letting you submerge. If you're not already too sleepy to dictate to your fancy, breathe slowly and deeply and imagine yourself in some favorite escapist setting . . . that appealing travel-folder beach in the sun country . . . the ideal meadow of your dreams, full of green and dew and bluebells . . . perhaps you see yourself in hacienda shade and a Mexican hammock, a place where all clocks have stopped . . . or a secret spot in a cool, dim, friendly forest where tall trees have made a clean pine-needle bed for you in a tiny clearing.

If it is night, and you are not entirely drowsy, when you get up you must move about very slowly and quietly. Think of yourself as a sleepwalker who must not be aroused or startled. Do nothing to break the spell.

CREATIVE SLEEP

It's possible to enhance the quality of your sleep and turn it into an effective ally of health and beauty.

If you experience sleep problems, devise a calming atmosphere before you go to bed. Be consciously involved and know you're preparing for a renewing experience; avoid serious conversations that stir up emotions before sleep. Forget the prototype Golden Anniversary couple ascribing marital and personal longevity to their always settling any quarrel just before tucking in. Don't take the chance. Nearly every sleep researcher has found that the most common cause of restless sleep is emotional turmoil. Give yourself the opportunity to be calmed down, not riled up.

BEFORE YOUR BEDTIME, VOLUMES—NOT VOLUME

I'm opposed to the ten- or eleven-o'clock news, and invite you to involve yourself during the hour immediately preceding sleep with creative, soothing pursuits. I personally have found this hour to be best for reading philosophy, feeling a direct link with the philosophers of long ago who spent sleepless nights just to consider the mysteries of the universe, the thoughts that I imprint into my consciousness as I fall asleep.

Keep a growth book at your bedside—poetry, the Bible, Marcus Aurelius, Lao-tzu—thoughts to put you into a comfortable frame of mind and lift you above petty worries and cares. The Golden Door weans away many insomniacs by providing every guest with nightstand copies of Erich Fromm's *The Art of Loving* and Paul Tillich's *The Courage to Be.*

TIPTOE THROUGH THE TRYPTOPHAN

If sleep still eludes you, the old remedy of warm milk is helpful for the very logical reason that milk contains the amino acid tryptophan, known for its mild sedative qualities. Heat the milk to hurry it into your system. This is an appropriate point for the progressive relaxation exercises. As I have said, you can conclude them with imagery, thinking of ocean water and gentle, swelling surf; or a plangent wind streaming through deep, sweet, yielding grass; or birds rising in almost effortless flight as if someone had just touched an antigravity button; or whatever imagery brings you peace.

At some time or other everybody wakens in the middle of the night. If your mind then insists upon wandering back to daytime cares, do sit up, turn on the light, and read a bit more.

HOW MUCH SLEEP DO YOU REALLY NEED?

Beware of excess sleep. Keep in mind that your metabolism slows down when you sleep. For that reason, over weeks, months, years, even a moderate eater can sleep herself into overweight. Also, too much sleep can make you feel sluggish and out of touch the next day. So, if you awaken feeling tired, it's usually another indication that more emphasis needs to be given to quality rather than to quantity.

After forty, you may find, as most people do, that you require less sleep every decade. Experiment. I find I do very well on six hours a night, and I love that extra hour to read, play, and do all the things I enjoy more than sleep.

According to a humorous old Irish adage, nature requires five hours of sleep; custom seven; laziness nine; and wickedness eleven.

Of course, the finest sleeping potion is contentment, pleasure in yourself and how you used each hour of the preceding day.

DREAMS AS FRIENDS AND TEACHERS

Since there are so many books about dreaming, this book won't go into the subject in any detail, except to say you'll probably rest better if you approach dream interpretation in the spirit of the Senoi people of Malaysia. The Senoi see their dreams as friends and teachers and are grateful for whatever comes to them in sleep. Why be upset if you can't figure out a dream, or if it casts you in a bad light? You provided the scenario, produced it, directed it, and acted in it. Don't be alarmed. Whatever the story line, it involved no real action or risk; you were in no physical danger.

The wakening brings you back to reality, and a bit of creative analysis may put the dream into perspective so that you may use it as a pathway to your own inner processes. Were you an observer? Was it uphill? There are many interesting books you may wish to research which will help you to use your dreams as a teaching tool. The triggering event is almost always an event of the preceding day, often in itself of little significance, but when it reverberates with something at a deeper level it can emerge into another level of consciousness as your dream.

YOUR DREAMS AS TRAINING FILMS

In the San Francisco area, dream workshops are an intriguing new development. Down in southern California, UCSD psychologist Ronald Lane believes that certain dreams—such as recurrent nightmares and threatening or unduly puzzling dreams—deserve a re-write. Dr. Lane guides his students in exerting a certain editorial control over their dreaming. His contention is that the observing self can put pressure to bear upon the participating dream self to buck up and show a little more starch in any terrifying situation. Other characters in your dreams, he admits, you may not have such success in directing. However, if a character has been menacing you in dream after dream, your observing self can prevail upon your participating self to be assertive, to ask the suspicious individual to identify himself and to admit precisely what skulduggery he is up to.

Part of the Lane system of dream control involves repeating just before going to sleep, ''I will remember my dream." This is especially indicated when you've had a vaguely troubling dream. Lane theorizes that you can rerun it in a clearer version, and have instant replay again next morning. Then you may want to subject your dream to professional analysis.

MEDITATION

Meditation may be vital to your survival. It well may turn out to be the best single means of avoiding future shock, of acting sensibly and selectively, and of guaranteeing your peace of mind. The time of simple activism is past. We no longer live in an orderly world where hard work and persistence and great deeds alone pay off. Nor is passivity an answer. Based upon both my own experience and witnessing the changes meditation has wrought in many of my guests, I'd say this discipline helps you along the route to the journey's end of this book: learning to live for *life.*

Meditation is the flip side of the mental process of thought. It's non-thought. When you think, you're systematically involved in construction work, like a child with building blocks. But in meditation, by using a variety of techniques, you can slow down your teeming brain and let it lie fallow. Your body needs to stop and start and stop again. So does your mind.

Most directions for meditation instruct you to find a comfortable sitting position, close your eyes, relax all your muscles, and think of nothing. Blot out all thoughts by concentrating upon your breathing. With each expiration you silently repeat a word. The word may be a mantra. The authors of *The Relaxation Response* suggest this simply be the word "one." They recommend that meditation be practiced no more than ten or twenty minutes daily, at least two hours after eating.

One technique of meditation involves focusing your mind on one object, such as a vase, or the bowl in the Japanese tea ceremony. After you have sat for a time, this simple and familiar container loses its everyday aspect. It looms unfamiliar and full of unrealized potential. This is the essence of meditation: It enables you to slip

---

outside your own mind and give your brain a half-turn, so you view yourself and the world from a new perspective, perceiving the same old things in a fresh way. Blake* caught it in his insightful stanza:

> To see a world in a grain of sand,
> And heaven in a wildflower,
> Hold infinity in the palm of your hand,
> And eternity in an hour.

STEPPING UP IN YOUR LIFE, NOT DROPPING OUT

Meditation is not withdrawal. It's an intuitive process, as opposed to the thinking process. You need not practice meditation in a vacuum any more than you have to leave the world behind you in order to do simple thinking. Rationality *and* intuition make fine companion tools for living.

Although millions have taken up meditation of one sort or another, it is still developing as a mass phenomenon. No one knows all the forms it may assume as it penetrates our culture. I'm convinced it will enhance our health. Explore: examine the many forms of meditation until you chance upon one giving you that feeling of coming home, a recognition that *this* is the one for you. But never stop looking and learning.

Should you find one book, one system, one master apparently supplying you with all the answers to the riddle of life, then heed the Zen parable: "If you meet a Buddha on the road, slay him!" This means that you must adhere to your own path of enlightenment and accept no gurus. Preserve your own subjective view of life. To find a pat system for coping with all of the world, man, and nature would simply be a denial of living and the beginning of death—for living is the process of growth and learning.

*William Blake (1757–1827), poet and mystic, a wonderful fellow who once penned the phrase "Energy is Eternal Delight."

DRUGS: THE TECHNOLOGY
OF SENSE MANIPULATION

We don't spend much time with prohibitions, since we're much more interested in determining what you should do than bothering about what you shouldn't. It's true, though, that the use of drugs such as alcohol, tobacco, mood pills, and coffee should be minimized in any sincere health plan. Moreover, even such medications as aspirin, antacids, sedatives, and any common painkiller can prevent body dialogue. They mask and make temporarily bearable conditions which should have prompt diagnosis and affirmative action by you and your physician. Take any medication only when the need is acute.

If you are a regular television watcher, you may find yourself persuaded that drugs of one kind or another are essential to everybody's happiness, success, and even survival. I asked a friend to monitor each of the commercial TV networks for one day. She filled pages with notes on headache pills, antacids, cold remedies, tonics, cures for the blahs, and the like. CBS led the misery parade with thirty-eight negative commercials in eleven and one-half hours; ABC was a nagging second with thirty-seven in ten hours; NBC clocked fifteen in eight hours. Your television set is telling you about three times an hour that there must be something wrong with you and that you'd better rush out and buy something for it.

THE WORLD IS READY
FOR THE UNADULTERATED YOU

It comes as no surprise to learn of experiments in which rats developed cancerous tumors when nitrites (nitrates and nitrites are in far too many commercially packaged meats, as the FDA has finally admitted) were combined with a tranquilizer and with a nonprescription sleeping aid (types of medication whose use has reached epidemic proportions).

Please note that I don't say all drugs should be eliminated totally. Alcohol in moderation is a pleasant and civilized way to augment a friendly occasion. At the Golden Door we occasionally use wine in our cooking and serve a glass of champagne on Saturdays to celebrate the termination of the week and the toasting of new friends. I do think a glass of white wine with friends is delightful as well as delicious; there's nothing very wrong with occasional social drinking—so long as it remains occasional. However, there is no doubt we would be better off if we eliminated all alcoholic beverages. Researcher Dr. Kenneth Lyons Jones of the UCSD Medical Center says there is no "safe dose" of alcohol for pregnant women. And in 1976 (these calculations are courtesy of *The Health Letter*), to cigarette smoking and excessive consumption of alcohol were attributable 25 percent of all this nation's direct costs of health care, or about $20.2 billion.

The time to cut back on all sorts of drug intake has arrived, not just because so many drugs are dangerous, but because all of them either lull, distort, or overly disturb your own awareness.

As one of my Golden Door friends says:

Every time I used to think I felt great, I was under the influence of one drug or another, some kind of phony thing. And when people would tell me to try healthful food or exercise or body awareness, I'd say, "Aah, I'd pull a muscle or break my neck or something. Leave me alone."

Now I want to keep forever this great feeling of being without an hallucinogen, valium, or anything like that.

She has recognized the incomparably heightened awareness that is the first step upward in consciousness raising and is also the foundation for a lasting sense of well-being.

SMOKE GETS IN YOUR EYES . . .

It also gets in your skin crevices, and other people's lungs and hair.

When cigarettes were popularized toward the end of the last century, young people who affected worldliness used to refer to them jocularly as "coffin nails," little guessing how appropriate that epithet might be.

I'm glad to report that social customs at last are being turned around. Grace Bechtold, my Bantam Books editor and a Golden Door guest, confirms that the habit of smoking is less and less socially acceptable. "I'm not as impressed by the arguments about health, since my health is okay. What's starting to get to me very badly is that smoking is becoming more and more repulsive to a lot of people. And who wants to be repulsive? To anybody?"

Not all friction is among business acquaintances. I overheard one guest tell another, "Since I gave up smoking I've had problems with my sex life. When I kiss my wife, it's like kissing an ashtray."

Here is a theory I intuited some time ago, before there was any scientific evidence at all: It would seem to me that each and every time one inhales tobacco smoke, the capillaries immediately affected are the ones adjacent to the nasal passages and to the brain. These thus receive a shade less of that most vital substance, oxygen. The idea is not so farfetched, since it's generally accepted that constriction of the capillaries is part of the effect of smoking. What an alarming thought, for within the brain lies our ability to live fully.

And now comes the *Brain Mind Bulletin* with an article headlined "Nicotine Can Cause Lasting Memory Deficit, Tests Show." This concerns a UCLA study, duly reported in the *American Journal of Psychiatry* by scientists from the Department of Psychology and Psychiatry. Testing was done on word recall. The non-nicotine group scored significantly higher than the nicotine smokers—and continued to score higher two days after the smoking experiment!

ARE YOU AN INVOLUNTARY SMOKER?

Although in some states smoking is being banned in public places, the rights of the nonsmoker are continually violated everywhere. An article in *Lancet* has theorized that one hour in a smoky room can be the equivalent of inhaling 15 cigarettes firsthand. Even if you aren't being stifled, if there's a smoker around you the chances are that you're breathing "side-stream smoke," more virulent even than "mainstream smoke." If you work closely with a pack-a-day smoker, you may even have traces of nicotine in your urine.

Saddest is the plight of child victims of inconsiderate smokers. A study made by James R. White, an exercise physiologist at UCSD Medical School, reports that secondhand smoke can elevate a child's blood pressure and heart rate.

TIPS TO HELP YOU QUIT SMOKING

If you feel you can't quit smoking overnight—and there are millions like you—perhaps one or some or all of the following five methods will help:

1. Make it inconvenient to smoke by keeping cigarettes in relatively inaccessible places.

2. Keep a log of each cigarette you smoke; note the time and the circumstances, as well as your emotional state.

3. Write down your reasons for wanting to quit; then remind yourself frequently of all the advantages of not smoking.

4. Consciously change all the habits and circumstances associated with the times you smoke.

5. When you have gradually but methodically cut down to one pack a day, you're ready to try the drastic plunge: cold turkey.

6. I have been telling my guests for years to follow a variation of this plan, an excellent system credited to Dr. Donald T. Frederickson: Whenever you buy a carton of cigarettes, wrap a piece of paper from a notepad around

each pack and secure with rubber bands. Every time you take out your pack for a smoke, write down the time of day and why you are having a cigarette. At day's end, grade the cigarettes you have smoked (Which did you most enjoy? Which did you seem to need most?), on a descending scale of one to five. After you finish a pack, file the slip of paper. Within a week or two, take out the file. Probably you will find written evidence that you already have achieved a real decrease in your smoking habit, simply because you have been accountable to yourself for each death-inducing drag. Then begin on the next step: eliminate all the smoking time periods scoring only four and five, which obviously were cigarettes you lit more automatically than enjoyably and should be able to give up with relative ease.

7. If you really want to kick the habit, and all else fails, check the Yellow Pages of your telephone directory and settle on one of the many peer-group therapy organizations that have good track records because they reflect some of the A.A. philosophy: Each fellow sufferer helps the other, and even the leader/teacher at one time was a victim, too.

A stop-smoking method to avoid is that called "stimulus satiation," in which for several minutes you rapidly puff on a cigarette. This speeds up breathing and heart rates, raises blood pressure, and worst of all blocks delivery of oxygen to vital tissues. The latter could be fatal.

A change of pace and place worked remarkably well for Calvin Klein, the fashion designer. Besides several annual ready-to-wear dress collections, Klein's imprimatur has been extended to nearly every branch of fashion—scarves, linens, suede and leather, and—currently—cosmetics. In addition to designing, he is an astute businessman, staying on top of all his company's recent expansions.

"It's normally a high-pressure business," says this three-pack-a-day man. "I work late a great deal of the time, and when we're setting up a show it's not unusual for me to work twenty-four hours without stopping."

One day he broke a promise to join friends on a trip

to South America. "It was going to be one of those twenty-four-hours-a-day partying trips. I didn't need that," says Klein, who engages in meditation and the study of mind control. Instead he went to Rancho La Puerta.

> I got up at six-thirty, climbed a mountain, breathed fresh air, ate healthful food, exercised, got a lot of sun and went to bed early. It was incredible! The second day, I didn't want a cigarette. And I didn't smoke again until I left after seven days. I had a sense of being healthy. I felt happy. It was the greatest.

HERE ARE SOME SMOKING STATISTICS MORE GRIM THAN VITAL

Americans smoked 603 billion cigarettes in 1975, an increase of 9 billion over the previous years. That represents 2.4 billion packs per month or an average of 11.2 cigarettes a day for every man and woman in the country over 18, according to the Annual Report of the Federal Trade Commission. U.S. statistics indicate that despite the increase in smokers, adult smokers are dwindling in increasing numbers, because they are proving themselves equal to the challenge of breaking the habit—certainly an encouraging example to the 95 percent of remaining smokers who tell the polls that they too would like to quit.

The real tragedy in the statistics is the revelation that young Americans are smoking even more heavily, and there is a sharp increase among teenage and even younger girls, according to William H. Foege, director for the Center for Disease Control in Atlanta. Foege advised the Senate Human Resources Subcommittee that more than 30 percent of boys and girls 17 and 18 have pretty well established the habit of smoking. Of course you have read of the health hazards to the child of the pregnant and, later, of the nursing mother. And now women have accumulated their own grim statistics on tobacco-related terminal cancer, heart disease, emphysema, and bronchitis.

Subliminal antismoking support is now coming from many sources, occasionally tripped up in unexpected quarters: According to a *Medical Tribune* survey, 78.7 percent of the physicians queried responded that they advise their patients to give up cigarettes, although 46.7 percent still permitted waiting-room smoking.

TAKING THE WRAPS OFF THAT SEDUCTIVE CIGARETTE PACKAGE

HEW Secretary Joseph Califano has announced that his department will lend a firmer hand by studying the matter of increased federal cigarette taxes, and by a sizable increase in federal funds spent on antismoking education. But the National Commission on Smoking and Public Policy would like HEW to go a lot further with antismoking education programs: with tighter restrictions on cigarette advertising; with a ban on classroom smoking by public-school students and teachers; with a more explicit warning on cigarette packaging; and, above all, with the phasing out of the price-support policy under which the federal government has annually spent millions of dollars to support tobacco. Why should tax dollars underwrite a crop which the AMA now tells us causes irreversible heart damage—and which the FTC admits produces carbon monoxide when smoked?

It took the AMA all this while to admit that smoking is bad for you. But now that Dr. Julius Richmond, the nation's top health officer, says there's no such thing as "tolerable levels" in certain low-tar brands of cigarettes, tobacco has been stripped of its last defensive smoke screen.

REALLY CARING ABOUT SKIN CARE

It's fitting to close a chapter on the body and all its senses by paying tribute to your skin, which packages everything so miraculously. Treat it tenderly.

Your skin is a fantastically intricate sensory receiver and transmitter—it advertises to the outside world your inner state.

If you want perfect skin, good heredity helps. There isn't a thing that you can do about your genes. But there's plenty you can do about exercise, the food you eat, and the water you drink. Carelessness in these crucial matters shows up in the skin more quickly than anywhere else.

Your delicate facial skin is constantly subjected to external irritations. Excessive wind and sun dry it. Smog and chemical wastes assail it. Ingredients contained in your own cosmetics may be assaulting it. Add to this the skin's own debris as it sheds cells and excretes sweat and oils, and you have a bothersome combination. Dead cells, when abandoned on the skin's surface, roll up inside any tiny creases. Removing this microscopic trash from your skin is what effective cleansing is all about.

Each person has, on the average, about two square yards of skin; it varies in thickness from one-thirty-second to one-eighth of an inch, and weighs about seven pounds. Each hardworking square inch harbors nearly twenty billion cells, six hundred fifty sweat glands, over two hundred fifty sensors for heat and cold and pressure, some one hundred sebaceous glands, seventy-eight nerves, twenty blood vessels and muscles.

Skin does so much more than cover you. It helps to regulate body temperature, excrete waste materials, and keep some fluids in and others out. It provides the sensory transition between you and the rest of the world.

Even if treated reasonably well, the skin is sure to lose some elasticity because of the normal thickening that comes with age. But given superlative care, your skin can better renew itself and stay young-looking longer.

CLEANSING AND CAMOMILE

Hungary has given the world many famous international beauties and professional beauty advisors. I am told this is due to the Hungarian woman's preoccupation with facial cleansing, simplified for her by the availability of good water and the tradition of using camomile, which has been valued as a complexion safeguard for thousands of years.

Because the sensitive skin can suffer broken capillaries if rubbed harshly with a washcloth, the Golden Door suggests using a water-soluble cleanser (not soap, which is high in alkalinity) that is removed with delicate little Italian sponges. This removes all except eye makeup, which should be taken off with camomile extract. Remove eye makeup with pieces of absorbent cotton torn to the size of small powder puffs. Do not buy the ready-made cotton balls, since they contain chemicals. Never substitute cleansing tissue, for it contains abrasive root particles.

Camomile can be bought in any health-food store that has a line of herb teas. Brew the camomile leaves as though preparing tea (buy the loose herb leaves, not the bags). You can soak your cotton eyepads in camomile and then put them on your eyes to relieve puffiness.

After you have applied the water-soluble cleanser, you will want to remove the residue left on your face. Again, employ your cotton puffs—twenty if necessary—after wetting them with a little water, followed by a skin freshener. In buying a freshener, look for one without alcohol if your skin is dry; as much as 8 percent alcohol may be suitable for some normal skin; a higher percentage of alcohol can be indicated if your skin is oily.

It is a good idea to search your face for whiteheads during the cleansing operation. Dab at them with Q-tips dipped in skin freshener.

(Of course, when I talk about facial care, I mean your face, throat, and neckline area.)

Never cleanse your face more than twice a day unless you have an oily complexion.

BEGIN YOUR GREAT DAY
IN THE MORNING

After morning cleansing, splash tepid or cool water on your face ten or fifteen times. Follow this by splashing with a skin refresher to close your pores and wake you up. Camomile will befriend you in the morning, too. Spray your face with mild camomile tea, which you have refrigerated in a spray bottle. Your face will be left soothed by an oily substance in the camomile. Don't let all the water evaporate. Leave enough dewy liquid on your skin so that moisture will be locked in when you apply a light moisturizing lotion as a protective base.

Last, to arm yourself against the day, use a good covering makeup foundation. Fortunately, these are once again in fashion. Fashionable or not, they are a protection and a necessity.

Besides your daily cleansing routine, you must add weekly ones. A facial sauna is a multi-purpose cleanser, loosening dead cells, purifying clogged pores, stimulating your skin's circulation, and providing the water your face needs in order to be smooth and young-looking. Again, rely on camomile leaves. A ten-minute camomile facial sauna will benefit every type of skin. You do not have to buy a facial-sauna machine. Substitute the old-fashioned pot-a-boiling on your stove top, and make a tent over it and your head with a large towel, but do be careful to turn the heat off after the water boils.

A mask is a weekly must as well—clay for cleansing, a gel or nondrying mask for moisturizing. If you, like most people, have a combination complexion—fairly oily on the forehead-and-nose T-zone but rather dry elsewhere—you will find it expeditious and doubly beneficial to use both types of mask at one time.

Another dividend-paying once-a-week ritual is the exfoliating mask or lotion, a gentle, invisible way to accelerate the removal of dead skin residue. It may show you that although the top layer of your skin appears dry, there is normal skin just beneath. More costly but worth considering is the rotating electric brush (of goat hair) for dusting off the shedding outer layer.

HOW TO USE THE CRÈME DE LA CREAM

You probably have already found a nourishing cream or a night cream that is compatible with your skin type. But the best beauty-care products in the world are not very good unless they are used properly. First of all, try to use one product line because the individual preparations are keyed to one another and can do their best work together.

Most people use more cream than is necessary. The skin can absorb only so much. If your skin is so dry that you feel the first thin application isn't sufficient, wait a bit and reapply. It's a good plan to cream your face after your nightly bath or shower, and then remove any excess before getting into bed. Your skin should breathe during the night.

An expert would vary some of the above advice according to the part of the world in which you live. In rain, for example, you would not need to use the richer of your two face creams. And if your home has air conditioning and/or steam heating, you will be wise to combat this drying effect by setting out several shallow bowls of water (so that the water evaporates) containing two little flowers—ideally, a Japanese flower arrangement very like those gracing each *tokonoma* at the Golden Door. This will help keep moisture in your skin.

SKIN CARE FOR MEN

You probably have heard the theory that the daily shave, which scrapes away a great many of the dead cells that cling to the face, is the reason many middle-aged men look younger than middle-aged women. But at the Golden Door we have demonstrated that men require more assiduous cleansing than women do. That's partly because men so far have neglected their complexions and partly because men have larger facial pores and oilier skin than women. This leaves them more susceptible to blackheads.

Although a lot of men still imagine there's something unmanly about complexion care, all would benefit from the use of a good water-soluble cleansing milk at least once a week. Our male guests at the Golden Door want to feel good and look good, and their built-in prejudice against skin care vanishes as their skin becomes positively clean.

Here's one last word of skin-care wisdom for both men and women: When leaving a swimming pool, always take care to thoroughly cleanse from your face the chlorine residue.

WATER WORKS WONDERS

Treat your skin to the widest possible range of water pressures and temperatures. Try this refresher: a long, steamy, hot bath with your favorite herbal scent to lull you into drowsiness, followed by a sudden splash of cool water to revive you. At some point during the bath, wake up your body (not your face) with a sponge-like loofah, or substitute a rough washcloth.

A fine all-over skin-awakener for your afterbath is to slap yourself briskly but lightly over your entire body with a cold wet washcloth. Or, with your hands cupped, rain light punches on your wet body from head to foot. And when you emerge from the bath, don't always coddle your skin with a velour towel if that's your custom. Use a rough Turkish or linen towel, snapping it strongly back and forth across your legs and bottom and back until the skin there is wake-up pink.

MUCH HUBBUB ABOUT A TUB

A big business in California and the west is the redwood hot tub, not for rub-a-dub-dub but for relaxation, and even for social relaxation. Because of California's reputation for a swinging life-style—and many photographs of mixed sexes *au naturel* (this common French phrase translates to mean both "naked" and "cooked plainly")—the rest of the country mistakenly equates the new hot tub with some kind of a sex trip. These tubs are equipped with heaters as well as circulating pumps. After twenty minutes to one hour of therapeutic temperatures of about 100 degrees, soakers are so relaxed they can't make conversation, let alone each other. Like the seagoing wooden shoe, the wooden tub is the perfect flagship for Wynken, Blynken, and Nod.

Pregnant women are cautioned to spend no more than five to seven minutes in these hot tubs.

I rely on a before-dinner swim or shower when I've had a particularly tiring day. I love the feeling of the water pouring down, washing away the day's accumulated tensions. Whenever I feel like a weary prune, water refreshes me, spruces me up, unwrinkles my senses, and perhaps gladdens the fish I once was.

SUN

Although recent warnings against excessive sunbathing have proliferated, it remains hard for some of us to believe anything that feels so good could do serious harm. But it does. Too much sun can cause skin cancer to develop later in life. At any stage, it ages your skin. Use common sense and don't permit temporary enjoyment of a deep tan to overrule your body's sense of what's good for it. The skin loses sensitivity as it darkens and thickens. Its ability to function diminishes. You can acquire a coat of leather if you sunbathe excessively. In the temperate zones, limit yourself to a maximum of twenty minutes of bright sunshine daily, fewer as you grow older.

Always use a sunscreen if you're in bright sunlight; if you are fair and susceptible to sunburn, use a stronger sun block on sensitive spots. Your pharmacist or cosmetician can suggest one.

AIR, YOUR PRIVATE
CRYSTAL OCEAN

During too much of your life, your skin surface is captive and unable to breathe—encapsulated within garments of various kinds. Moisture can't evaporate. Oxygen and sunlight, germ-killers supreme, can't approach the skin. This perpetual covering fosters a welcoming environment for fungi and bacteria. For half an hour or so every day, go barefoot and as nearly nude as you can.

Don't be overprotective of your skin when in the atmosphere of your bedroom. Sleep bare. Let your body be on intimate terms with the climate, the temperature, and the humidity.

There's an internal thermometer in our bodies, but like many other physical abilities, our capacity to regulate our temperature will atrophy if we don't make use of it. That is why I'm opposed to the electric blanket. It hampers your body's ability to respond to communications from your closest environment.

Whether you dress in jeans or a garment with a Bill Blass label is not important. What is important, however, is how well you fit into nature's undergarment—that exquisitely sheer original, your own body. Take care of it. Surround yourself with pure air whenever possible. And treat yourself to great drafts of fresh air with a minute or two of deep breathing several times a day. It's not enough to develop your breathing capacity through cardiovascular activity. A deadline situation or some such crunch, a flash of resentment, or a heated exchange of words, all these produce tensions that can constrict breathing without your even being aware of it. That's when a minute or two of deep breathing exerts its head-clearing, tension-dispelling effect. Inhale slowly through your nostrils, filling first your abdominal cavity, then your rib cage, *then* your lungs. Exhale slowly. Keep your posture very straight throughout. You'll not only feel better, you'll *be* better.

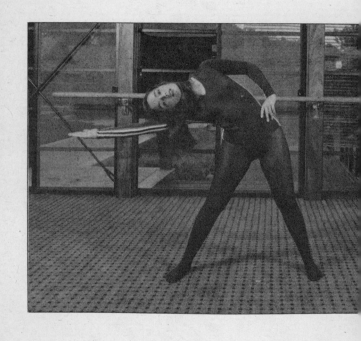

CHAPTER IV

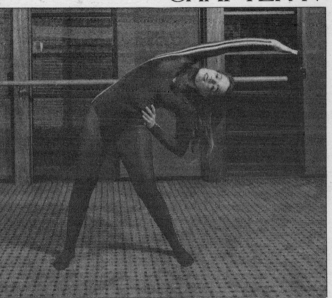

GOLDEN DOOR
PRE-ANYTHING
EXERCISES
(For Stretching, Strengthening, and Limbering Plus Body Talk for Precision Trimming)

You've paid for this book a very small percentage of what a week at the Golden Door costs. To make it worthwhile, you will have to supply a missing ingredient: yourself. Yourself on the exercise mat. Walking and jogging. Laughing and feeling better than ever before.

All Golden Door guests arrive on Sunday, realizing full well they are sentencing themselves to eleven-hour activity days devoted to renewing their minds and bodies, and that much of the time will be passed at hard labor. All ages, from teenager to young-at-eighty, are attracted to this goal.

On the first morning and every day thereafter, they receive a personalized daily activity schedule. The number of class periods is always the same, but the duration and intensity are influenced by the individual's level of fitness and goals for the week. Here is a typical daily schedule:

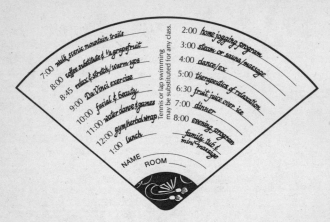

When the guests leave the Golden Door a week later, they take with them the sum of what the instructors and I can impart to them (and what I'm striving so hard to put in this book), the encouraging example of what they have achieved in one week, the resolve to apply all this to daily living. With them go their new ABC's, which the President's Council on Physical Fitness and Sports proposes so well:

1. A regular exercise schedule
2. Supplementary physical recreation
3. Stepped-up ordinary physical activity
4. Physical activity in the day's occupation

DESIGN YOUR
OWN GOLDEN DOOR
EXERCISE PLAN

The Golden Door judges its success by how well departing guests sustain their exercise high and integrate a regular exercise program into their own life-style. Most returnees gratify us. Some even astonish us. These are the people who use their first Golden Door week as a departure point for all sorts of self-realization.

When our guests leave, they take with them two cassettes, one for relaxation, and the other individually designed for the guest's own at-home exercise program.

Set against soothing, undemanding, fantasy-inspiring music, the relaxation or sleep cassette contains apropos quotations, relaxation techniques, relaxation countdown, and self-hypnosis hints. Many guests use their tape to further unwind after twilight exercise routines. Others listen with earphones, in order not to disturb one's bed partner.

THOSE WHO MAKE THEIR OWN TAPE STICK WITH IT

With a background of light rock music characterized by a strong back beat, the exercise cassette is one which has been worked out by the guest and the Golden Door cassette exercise specialist jointly. Once home, the guest often is inspired to write us rapturous reports about the cassette and the results obtained. Besides being brightly evocative of Golden Door atmosphere and expertise, the tape settles for each guest the nagging question of what exercises to do at a session, in what sequence, and for how long.

This is easy enough for you to do as well. Set aside a quiet hour with this book in hand, a pad and a pencil, and a full-length mirror. You also will need a cassette player, a blank thirty-minute tape, and a phonograph or a second cassette player stocked with favorite music.

Look long at yourself, nude, in the mirror. Next, imagine that you are the exercise specialist at the Golden Door about to prescribe for you which exercises you should do and the number of times you should do them. In succession, be the scriptwriter as you put the exercises in sequence; the music arranger as you select the right tempos.

BE YOUR OWN CHORUS LINE

That done, with script in hand and thirty minutes of happy-making music on your phonograph, talk yourself through your first exercise-program production, including warm-ups and cool-downs. Your tape will obviate the need to remember what action comes next, and instead will allow you to think about the feeling of movement within your body. As you become more expert you'll find you want to change your program. Where do you obtain additional exercise instructions? There are so many good books on the subject. Bonnie Prudden has written several. *Miss Craig's 21-Day Shape-Up Program for Men and Women* (Random House, 1968) is an excellent standard stocked by most libraries. As you become adept and wish something more advanced, you will learn much from the work of Nicholas Kounovsky.

Before you settle on any group of exercises, always check the dos and don'ts (pages 170-73), and keep them firmly in mind. For the beginner, the most important thing is beginning stretching, to warm and relax the muscles so they can perform easily and painlessly. If you are unaccustomed to any exercise, for the first week or so do the stretches only. Save the old tapes for reference; track your own trajectory in the fitness orbit.

You'll love being a cassette choreographer. To make your first tape, start with the Golden Door Pre-Anything Exercises.

THE GOLDEN DOOR
PRE-ANYTHING EXERCISES

It is said that 80 percent of the back trouble in the United States is caused by lack of exercise. But weakness is not confined to the old. If you've been inactive, your back may have grown weaker than you suspect.

To eliminate early-week soreness in the back and other parts of the body, the Golden Door sends its prospective guests a set of conditioners and back strengtheners to practice before checking in. Then, at the outset of the new guests' first week, a class is held to help ensure that guests do not strain their backs through overdoing or lack of condition.

Our guests have been so grateful for this innovation.

REMEMBER THAT YOUR MUSCLES CAN BE CAPRICIOUS

Never assume that you have advanced beyond the need for slow, gentle, unbouncy stretches, back strengtheners, and warm-ups. Professionals know better. Exercise instructors, ballet dancers, and others who practice daily disciplined movement are keenly aware how variable a thing is the flexibility of a muscle. From one day to the next it may tense and tighten.

Pre-Anything Exercises can take you safely into jogging, jumping rope, swimming, taking off for skiing, tennis, or whatever.

STRETCHES THAT FLOW:
back-strengthening and flexibility

This series of twenty-five exercises will give
your body a very thorough stretch.

ONE

a Lie flat on back, with arms at 90-degree angle to body, palms down. Feet are hips' width apart. Inhale as you draw up your legs, bending knees and placing soles of feet firmly on floor.

b Exhale slowly, and initiate movement in pelvis, lifting it forward as you roll up spine and lift torso from floor. Be careful *not* to arch back. Make your body, collarbone to knees, a straight line. Hold for count of 10 while you conclude exhale breath. As you progress, gradually increase count.

c Relax, inhale, and slowly roll spine back down to original position. Feel each vertebra touch floor.

d Perform 5 times. Gradually increase.

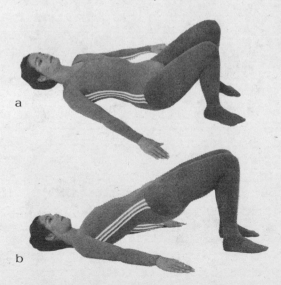

TWO

a Lie flat on back, with arms parallel to each other and resting on floor above head; palms upward. Feet are hips' width apart. Inhale as you draw up your legs, bending knees and placing soles of feet firmly on floor.

b Exhale slowly and initiate movement in pelvis, lifting it forward as you roll up spine and lift torso from floor. Be careful *not* to arch back. Make your body a straight line from collarbone to knees. Hold for count of 10 while you complete exhale breath. As you progress, gradually increase count.

c Relax, inhale, and slowly roll spine back down to original position. Feel each vertebra touch floor.

d Perform 5 times. Gradually increase.

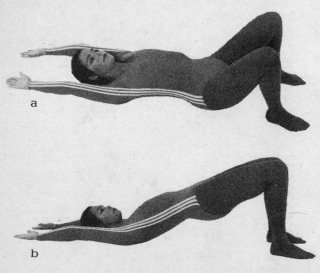

a

b

THREE

a Lie flat on back. Extended arms are against floor at right angles to body. Feet are six inches apart. Palms upward.

b Inhale as you draw up legs and clasp knees with hands.

c Exhale as you lock fingers. Press lower back into floor as you keep knees bent, and roll up spine, pulling knees toward you as if you were going to kiss them. Hold for count of 10 as you complete the exhale breath. As you progress, gradually increase count.

d Relax, inhale; and roll spine back down to original position, as you exhale once more.

e Perform 5 times. Gradually increase.

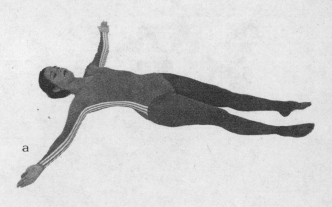

a

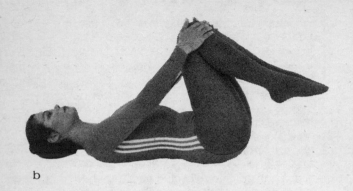

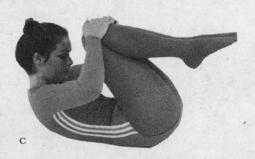

FOUR

a Lie flat on floor. Feet are six inches apart.
  Extended arms are against floor and at right
  angles to body; palms downward.

b Inhale as, flexing right foot and keeping knee
  straight, you raise right leg. Left leg should be
  relaxed, knee bent.

c Swing right leg toward left side, and touch
  foot to floor, as close to left palm as possible.
  Press right shoulder to floor, and exhale as
  you hold position for count of 15.
  (If you feel discomfort when you press down
  shoulder, at first simply relax shoulder.) As
  you progress, gradually increase count to 20,
  then to 25.

d Inhale as you lift right leg with straight knee.

e Relax and inhale as you return to original
  position.

f Reverse. Perform 5 times, each side.
  Gradually increase.

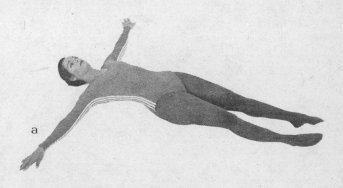

a

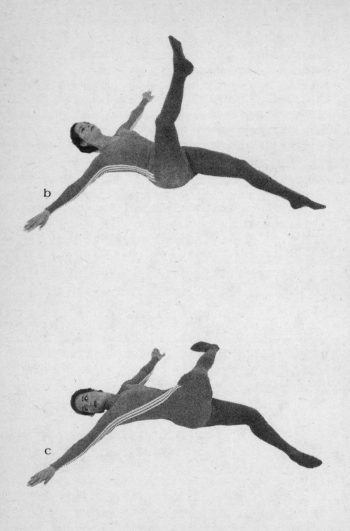

FIVE

a Lie on stomach. Arms rest on floor above head, elbows bent, palms down.

b Inhale as you lift left leg in back of you. Left knee is slightly bent. Do *not* arch back. Keep pelvic bone down.

c Hold for count of 5 while you exhale. As you progress, gradually increase count.

d Continuing to exhale, relax and return to original position.

e Reverse. Perform 5 times, each side. Gradually increase.

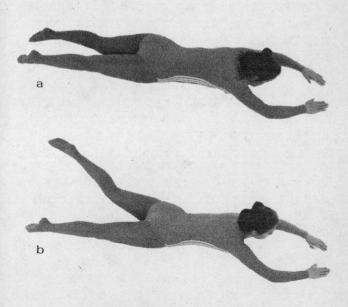

a

b

SIX

a Lie on stomach, with arms near sides, elbows slightly bent; palms up.

b Inhale as you extend right arm (elbow straight) and lift left leg. At same time, lift head while continuing to look down at floor.

c Hold for count of 5 while you exhale. As you progress, gradually increase count.

d Continuing to exhale, relax and return to original position.

e Reverse. Perform 5 times, each side. Gradually increase.

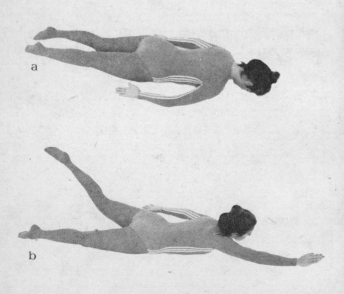

SEVEN

a Lie on back, with feet hips' width apart, soles of feet on floor. Arms on floor, at 90-degree angle to body; palms up.

b Inhale as you lift legs till they are at right angles to floor. Grasp backs of legs with both hands. Exhale as you

c Pull up torso. Roll up spine while drawing hands upward along the backs of your legs. Make sure legs keep their 90-degree angle. Do *not* pull them toward torso. Chin should be well tucked into chest.

d Hold for count of 5 while continuing to exhale. As you progress, gradually increase count.

e Relax, and roll spine back down to original position.

f Perform 5 times. Gradually increase.

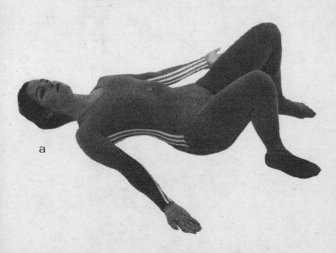

a

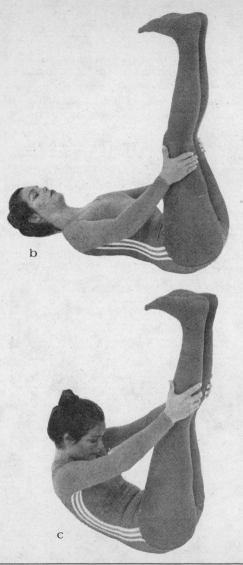

b

c

EIGHT

a Lie on stomach, legs straight, feet six inches apart. Head rests on floor, chin forward. Hands, palms up, are placed on each side of spine at midback; upper arms rest on floor.

b Inhale as you lift head while continuing to look down at floor.

c Hold for count of 5. As you progress, gradually increase count.

d Exhale as you relax and return to original position.

e Perform 5 times. Gradually increase.

When you have become proficient in this exercise, advance to variation:

a same as above

b Inhale slowly as you raise head and shoulders, taking care as you tilt back head, vertebra by vertebra.

c etc.

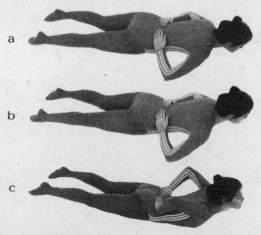

a

b

c

NINE

a Lie on stomach, feet are hips' width apart. Elbows are bent, palms turned to floor near shoulders.

b Inhale slowly as you straighten elbows, lift upper torso; take care as you tilt back head, vertebra by vertebra.

c Hold for count of 5, while you complete inhale breath. As you progress, gradually increase count.

d Exhale and relax, returning to original position.

e Perform 5 times. Gradually increase.

N.B.: If you have any lower-back problems, don't attempt this exercise.
Whenever you do perform Exercise 9, be sure to follow it immediately with Exercise 10, to rest spine.

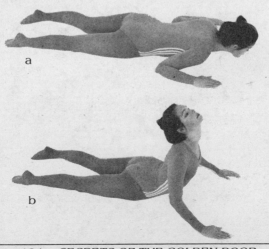

a

b

TEN

a Kneeling on floor, sit on your heels. Exhale
  as you bend forward, with parallel arms held
  straight, elbows resting near head. Palms
  downward.

b Inhale as you use your hands to "walk"
  away from your torso as far as you can, to
  ensure fullest stretch. Arms remain parallel to
  each other, elbows gradually straighten. Hold
  for count of 10. Gradually increase to 20,
  then to 25.

c Exhale as you bring your arms beside your
  body, palms upward. Head still rests against
  floor as you relax for count of 10.

d Perform 5 times. Gradually increase.

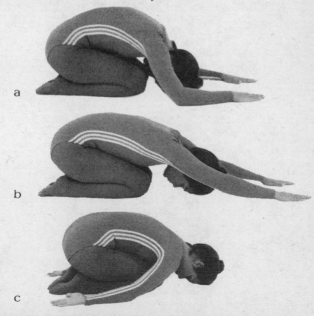

ELEVEN

a Kneeling on floor, sit on your heels. Pulling your shoulders down, make a very straight back.

b Still keeping a straight back, inhale as you clasp hands behind you.

c Exhale as you bend forward, dropping head to floor. Hands remain clasped. Push arms (straight elbows) up behind your head as far as you can.

d Inhale as you hold for count of 5. As you progress, gradually increase count.

e Exhale as you roll spine back up and return to kneeling position.

f Perform 5 times. Gradually increase.

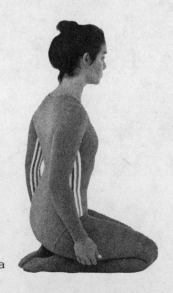

a

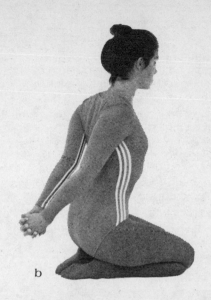

b

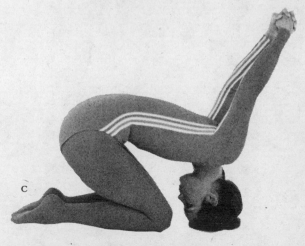

c

TWELVE

a Stand straight and tall, with feet planted directly under each hip. Knees should not be locked but relaxed—even slightly bent. Inhale as you stretch, parallel arms above head.

b Continue to exhale and inhale naturally as you imagine that there is a rope above you, its end just barely reachable. Very slowly, stretching first one arm and then the other, pretend you are pulling the rope down.

c Relax, and return to original position after you have ''pulled the rope down.''

d Perform 5 times with each arm. Gradually increase.

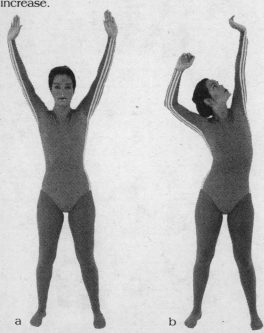

a   b

THIRTEEN

a Stand straight and tall, with feet planted directly under each hip. Knees should not be locked but relaxed—even slightly bent. Inhale as you reach up, stretching arms parallel above head. Interlock fingers, palms outward, directly above head, and

b Exhale as you stretch arms up and pull head down. Hold for count of 10. Gradually increase count.

d Relax head, and return to original position.

e Perform 5 times. Gradually increase.

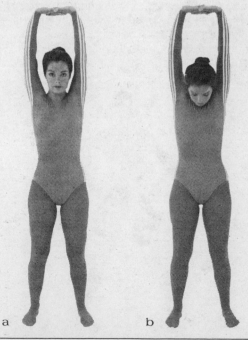

a   b

FOURTEEN

a Stand straight with feet wide apart. Knees should not be locked but relaxed—even slightly bent. Hands on hips.

b Inhale and exhale naturally as, first, you leave right hand on right hip and bend torso toward left side, extending left arm (elbow straight) parallel to floor—toward the left. Keep shoulders back. Palm of extended left hand is upward.

c Still holding right hand on right hip, in a rotary sweep bring both torso and left arm toward the front, and

d Continue rotary sweep as you bring torso to left side (also incline head to left), with left arm lifted above head.

e Relax, and return to original upright position.

f Reverse. Perform 5 times, each side. Gradually increase.

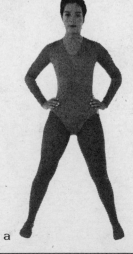

a

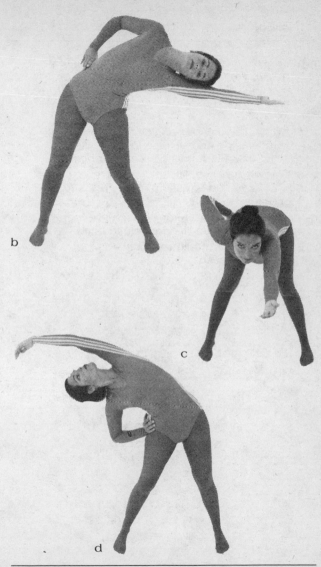

b

c

d

FIFTEEN

a Stand with feet wide apart. Knees are slightly bent. Arms are raised above head with hands curved inward—similar to ballet's fifth position. Exhale as you bend forward and relax arms.

b Slowly inhale as you dangle hands over floor toward left side and lift torso toward left, still keeping extended arms parallel near head.

c Still slowly inhaling, lift torso upward on left side till extended arms form right angles to floor. Pause to exhale.

d Inhale as you return to original upright position, and again lift arms above head.

e Reverse. Perform 5 times, each side. Gradually increase.

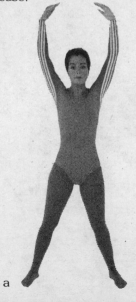

a

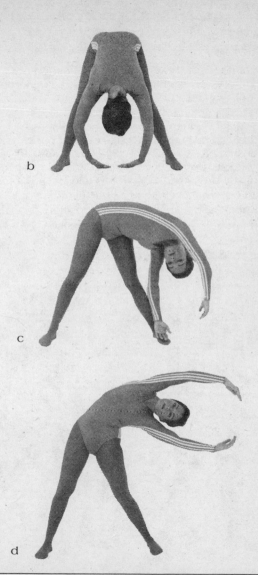

b

c

d

SIXTEEN

a Stand with feet wide apart, toes turned out. Elbows are slightly bent. Hands, held in front of body, are curved inward.

b Exhale as you bend knees, with hands placed on thighs midway above knees. Pelvis is slightly tilted. Do *not* arch back; hold it straight. (Even if you consider yourself flexible, do *not* bend so deeply that end of spine drops below knees.) Hold for count of 10; gradually increase count to 15.

c Inhale as you rise to original position.

d Perform 5 times. Gradually increase.

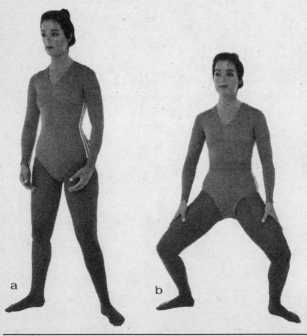

SEVENTEEN

a Stand with feet hips' width apart. Toes point straight ahead. Exhale completely as you bend forward from the waist, with bent knees. Relax arms completely, allowing hands to dangle. Head hangs heavily.

b Inhale as you initiate movement in pelvis and begin to roll spine back up to standing position, one vertebra at a time. Knees remain bent. Shoulders and head are the last to be lifted upright.

c Perform 5 times. Gradually increase.

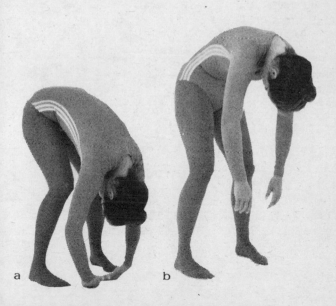

a   b

EIGHTEEN

a Stand with feet wide apart, toes straight ahead. Elbows are slightly bent. Hands, held in front of body, are curved inward.

b Exhale as you bend forward from torso, at same time taking a lunging step forward with left foot. Drop hands, palms down, to floor in front of you. (Hands should be somewhat more than your shoulders' width apart.)

c On the final exhale breath, drop onto bended right leg and crouch. Only ball of left foot rests on floor. Left toe should line up with right knee. Head should be relaxed.

d Inhaling, drop heel of left foot to help straighten yourself as you rise to starting position.

e Reverse. Perform 5 times, each side. Gradually increase.

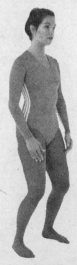

a

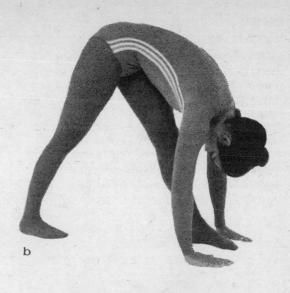

b

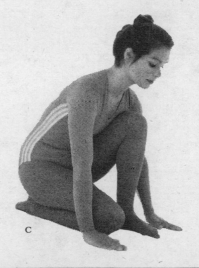

c

NINETEEN

a Sit on floor. (Sit forward, *not* on tailbone.) Spine must be straight. Inhale as you grasp ankles with your hands and press soles of feet together.

b Exhale as you bend forward to touch head to feet while bringing them as close to the crotch as possible. Really concentrate on tightening stomach muscles as you

c Inhale, and return to original sitting position.

d Perform 5 times. Gradually increase.

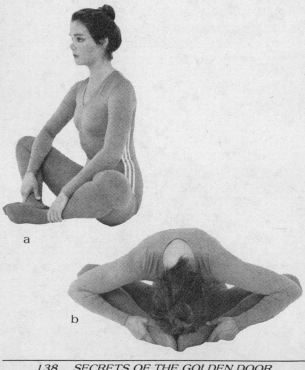

a

b

TWENTY

a Sit on floor, with good posture. Legs are
  straight. Feet, about six inches apart, are
  flexed.
b Try to keep back straight as you exhale and
  bend forward. Grasp flexed feet with both
  hands. Try to pull feet toward you. Let head
  relax. Hold for count of 10. Gradually
  increase.
c Inhale as you return to original sitting
  position.
d Perform 5 times. Gradually increase.

When you have become proficient in this
exercise, advance to this variation:

a same as above
b Bend forward as you exhale. Round back
  and relax head forward, touching it to knees.
  Hold for count of 5. Gradually increase.
c etc.

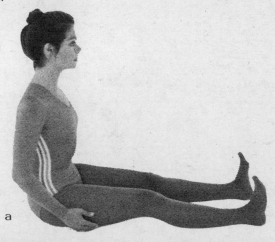

a

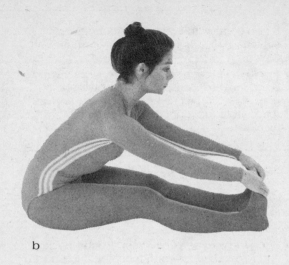

b

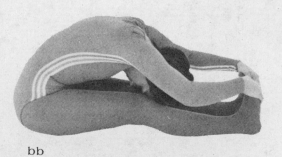

bb

TWENTY-ONE

a Sit on floor. Bend right knee and bring right leg behind you (try to bring right foot as close to right buttock as possible). Left leg with straight knee remains on floor in front of you. Flex left foot.

b Exhale as you bend forward and grasp left foot with both hands. Let head relax. Hold for count of 10. Gradually increase count.

c Inhale as you roll spine back up to sitting position.

d Reverse. Perform 5 times, each side. Gradually increase.

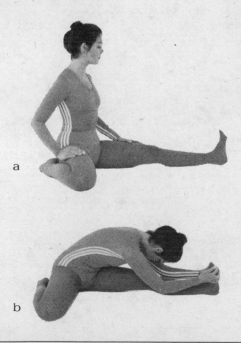

a

b

TWENTY-TWO

a Lie on floor on right side, with head resting on right hand. Hold bent left arm (palm down) in front of you, for balance.

b Inhale, and grab left foot with left hand. Attempt to press left heel into left buttocks. Tilt pelvis slightly forward at the same time, and incline left pelvic bone toward right. Keep right knee relaxed (this will eliminate strain on back). Hold for count of 10. Gradually increase count.

c Exhale as you relax and return to original position.

d Reverse. Perform 5 times, each side. Gradually increase.

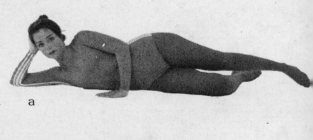

a

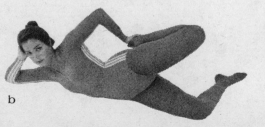

b

TWENTY-THREE

a Stand with feet wide apart, knees slightly bent. Exhale slowly as you bend forward halfway from waist. Hold both arms (elbows stiff) straight in front of you. Arms and torso are parallel with floor. Head is lifted so you can look at arms. Keep back flat.

b On final exhale, drop torso forward and clasp ankles with hands. Still keep back straight.

c Inhale as you round back and roll spine back up to standing position.

d Repeat 5 times. Gradually increase.

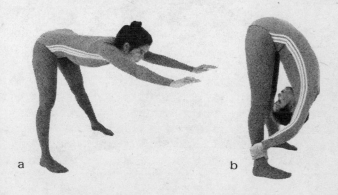

a   b

TWENTY-FOUR

a Sit on floor, spreading legs as widely as you can. Knees are straight, feet flexed. With elbows slightly bent, drop hands to floor in front of you.

b Exhale as you straighten arms, holding them parallel and reaching them out as far as possible in front of you, palms down on floor. Keep back straight.

c Inhale as you roll spine back up to original sitting position.

d Perform 5 times. Gradually increase.

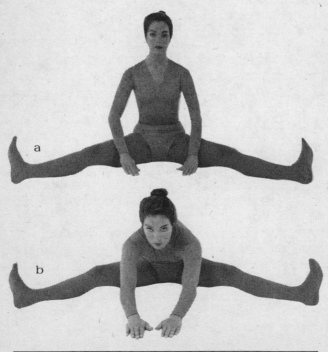

TWENTY-FIVE

a Stand straight, with legs far apart. Arms are straight out at sides, at right angles to body.

b Exhale, bending to left side, placing left hand on side of left thigh and letting hand slip down side of leg as torso bends. Right arm, elbow straight, is raised above head.

c Inhale, and return to upright position.

d Reverse. Perform 5 times, each side. Gradually increase.

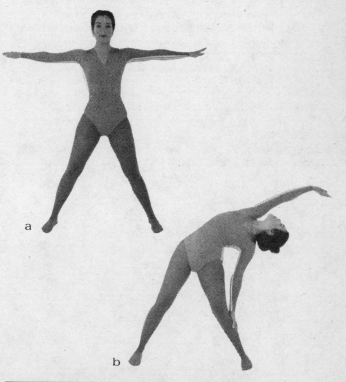

a

b

THE GOLDEN DOOR
BODY-TALK EXERCISES

These and all exercises you will perform to music. Pick persuasive, can't-be-ignored melodies with a clear happy beat. They inspire movement. You know how a child dances when music is played. Let the child within you emerge as you too dance about your room.

Spend time selecting the music you enjoy. (And whatever loose, comfortable clothing you choose for exercising, let it be happy-colored!) You should feel the melody even in your fingertips. Each morning at the Golden Door starts off with a familiar record, ''I Want to Teach the World to Sing.'' Whenever our guests hear it, as with a conditioned reflex, they begin to move.

Exercise mats aren't essential but they are certainly nice to have. A folded blanket will do as a substitute. The soft rug in your personal retreat is ideal.

The Golden Door often uses hula hoops, jump ropes, plastic balls (ten to twelve inches in diameter), balloons, and one-inch doweling rods approximately forty-five inches long. Yet Body-Talk Exercises have been designed for you to do without any equipment whatever.

Now that you've pre-exercised for exercise, you're ready to start Body Talk at an easy pace, and to savor every move you make!

ONE

BENEFIT: For stomach and waistline. Also good for lower back.

a Lle on back, arms flat on floor and at right angles to body; palms up. Knees bent, feet about six inches apart. Inhale and exhale with deep breaths as

b With knees still bent, press shoulders to floor, and try to keep feet in original position as you move both knees toward right, with right knee touching floor.

c Reverse, and continue rhythmical movement from side to side. Touch 10 times, each side. Gradually increase.

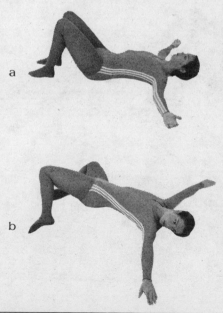

TWO

BENEFIT: For stomach.

a Lie on back and inhale. Arms are clasped behind head. Feet are hips' width apart, with knees bent. Soles are on floor.

b Exhale, and raise left knee and right elbow to meet each other. It is important that they touch directly over the waistline.

c As you inhale, relax and return to original reclining position.

d Reverse. Perform 5 times, each side. Gradually increase.

N.B. Repetitions should be slow and controlled.

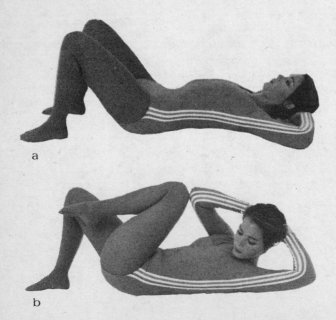

a

b

THREE

BENEFIT: For buttocks and inner and outer thighs.

a Lie on left side; left knee is bent. Rest head on left hand (left elbow bent). Right elbow is bent, and right palm on floor in front of you aids balance. Right knee rests on floor, and lower part of right leg is perpendicular to floor.

b Inhale as you straighten right knee and flex right foot while lifting right leg. How high you lift is not important.

c Exhale, and return to original reclining position.

d Reverse. Repeat 5 times, each side. Gradually increase.

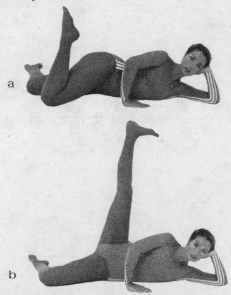

A VARIATION ON NO. 3

BENEFIT: For buttocks and outer thighs. Also stomach.

a Same starting position as above.

b Inhale as you bring right knee forward. At the same time, right arm goes back in opposite direction, straightening elbow. Head turns to watch movement of right arm.

c Exhale while rolling torso slightly to right. Bent left arm, with palm now turned to floor, supports you as extended right arm (elbow stiff) reaches forward, hand touching floor. Head turns to watch right arm. At same time, you lift right leg behind you.

d Relax, inhale, and return to original starting position.

e Reverse. Repeat 5 times, each side. Gradually increase.

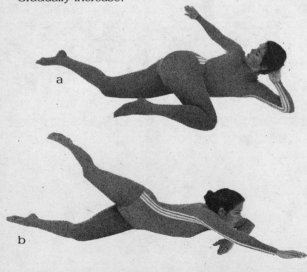

FOUR

BENEFIT: For buttocks and inner thighs.

a Almost same starting position as above, but left leg is straight. Right leg, with bent knee, rests on floor in front of you.

b Inhale as you lift left leg behind you, keeping both knee and foot flexed. Hold for count of 5. Gradually increase.

c Exhale, as you return to original position.

d Reverse. Perform 5 times, each side. Gradually increase.

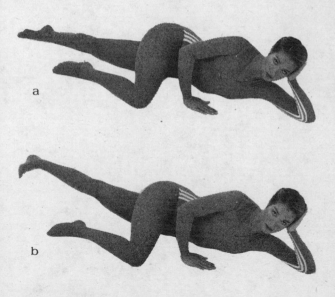

FIVE

BENEFIT: Buttocks, inner thighs, stomach.

a Similar starting position to above, but head goes down one level, no longer supported by bent left arm, which now rests on floor in front of you, palm down, for balance. Left knee is bent. Right leg is in front of you, foot flexed.

b With foot still flexed, inhale as you lift right leg off floor. Hold for count of 5. Gradually increase.

c Exhale and return to original reclining position.

d Reverse. Perform 5 times, each side. Gradually increase.

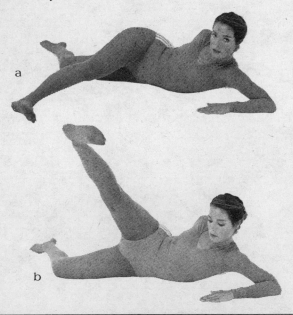

SIX

BENEFIT: Pectorals, upper arms, and flabby back area around underarms.

a Stand with feet about six inches apart. Bend over and try to make an absolutely horizontal line with your torso back and neck. Watch your arms dangle with palms turned in.

b Keeping back, knees, and elbows straight, inhale as you lift arms at your sides and pull them back as far as you can.

c Exhale, and return to original position.

d Perform 5 times. Gradually increase times and speed.

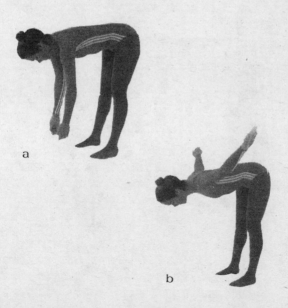

a

b

SEVEN

BENEFIT: Pectoral muscles and upper arms.

a Stand with feet hips' width apart, knees bent. Arms are extended at shoulder level, at right angles to sides of body.

b Holding arms high and elbows stiff, make quick scissors movements with arms as you pass your right hand over your left, then your left over your right, etc. Move straight arms no farther than you must to make the quick changeover.

c Perform 5 sets, left and right. Gradually increase times and speed.

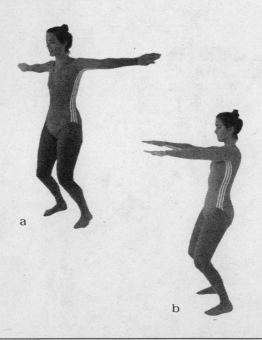

a

b

EIGHT

BENEFIT: Pectorals, upper arms, and flabby back area around underarms.

a Stand with feet about six inches apart, knees bent. Arms at sides.

b Keeping back straight and elbows stiff, and still presenting palms of your hands toward rear, inhale and raise arms in back of you as high as you can. Hold for count of 5.

c Exhale, and return to original position.

d Perform 10 times. Gradually increase.

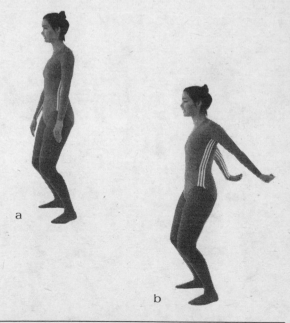

NINE

BENEFIT: Pectorals, upper arms, and flabby back area around underarms.

a Stand with feet hips' width apart, knees slightly bent. Hold upper arms at level with shoulders, at right angles to sides of body. Drop lower left arm, and at same time inhale, turn head to right and look at your lower right arm as you point it upward. Then, quickly, exhale as you

b Turn head to left and look at your lower left arm as you point it upward; lower right arm points down.

c Perform 5 times, each side. Gradually increase.

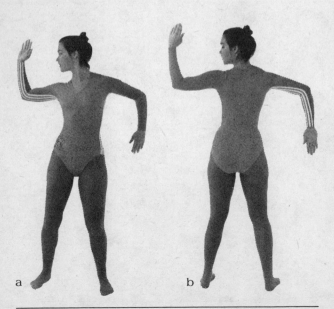

a   b

TEN

BENEFIT: Pectoral muscles.

a Stand with feet hips' width apart, knees slightly bent. Fold arms away from body at shoulder level. Right hand grasps outside of lower left arm; left hand grasps inside of lower right arm. *Be sure to keep your shoulders down in back* as you inhale and push hands away from each other while continuing to grasp arms. Then quickly exhale, and push hands toward each other— still holding onto your arms. (This is a lovely near-secret exercise you can resort to at random moments nearly everywhere, as you literally "shoot your cuffs.")

b Alternate by switching hand position. Repeat 5 times, each side. Gradually increase.

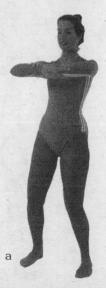

a

ELEVEN

BENEFIT: Pectorals, upper arms, and flabby back area around underarms.

a Stand with feet hips' width apart. Raise right arm, pointing elbow upward; dropping lower right arm behind your back. Bent left arm is behind you.

b Palm upward, upper left arm reaches up right shoulder; left elbow is at mid-back. Hook righthand fingertips over lefthand fingertips. Inhale, and with fingers holding firmly, try to pull hands apart. Hold for count of 5, and exhale.

c Reverse. Perform 5 times, each side. Gradually increase.

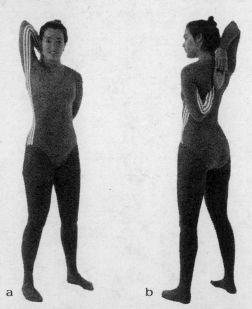

a   b

TWELVE

BENEFIT: Shoulder muscles.

a Stand with feet about six inches apart. Arms at sides. Bring shoulders forward as you inhale and lift them as if to touch your ears.

b Still hunching shoulders high, roll them toward your back.

c Bring shoulders down in back on the exhale, and repeat cycle. Perform shoulder rolls 5 times, then reverse sequence by making it back-to-front, instead of front-to-back.

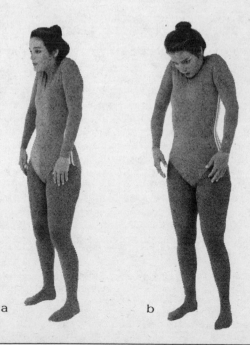

a   b

HOW TO SPEAK BODY TALK

You must believe me when I say that your body is communicating with you all the time. Unfortunately, most humans in civilized societies have simply fallen out of the habit of listening.

Simple biofeedback techniques could help you relearn how to interpret your body's urgent messages to you, and how to relay effective messages of your own. First, biofeedback instrument readout would graphically show you what your body is saying. In the second step, you would see your body reaction when you "speak" directly to its parts. One of the first common demonstrations consists of your telling your thumb that it is growing very warm. Shortly, the little thermometer which has been attached would begin to show your thumb temperature rising.

YOUR OWN ACTION HOT LINE

See for yourself, sometime when your hands are cool or at normal temperature: tell one thumb that the weather is tropical, that despite the heat you are placing your thumb near a roaring blaze, that you're holding a teacup handle which almost burns.

The implicit lesson in this early step in biofeedback training you can easily convert to your own benefit in an exercise period, without need of machinery.* Begin by zeroing in on one muscle at a time, feeling that you really are "getting inside" the muscle, telling it how it is becoming very, very warm and pliable. It is in relaxation classes that Golden Door guests first pick up this easy technique, and you may wish to try it first with one of the basic Pre-Exercises above. Too, you can insert it into Body-Talk Exercises, which also are extremely easy to follow.

*As Dr. Alyce Green of the Menninger Foundation (Topeka, Kansas) confirms: "Biofeedback instruments are just sophisticated mirrors that show us how we are doing when we try to make certain changes; and when we know how to make the changes we don't need the mirrors anymore."

IT'S LIKE SLIPPING
INTO YOUR OWN BODY

At each stage of an exercise, try to keep your mind focused on the part of the body which is receiving the benefit. Mentally blanket that area as if your body were concentrating all its healing power right there. Of course, you also are to accompany your mental body talk with a strong message of love. (If plants can respond to human affection, can your own body do less?)

Once you catch onto the easy but quite revolutionary Body-Talk principle, you will never again want to exercise with a distracted mind.

And as you gain Body-Talk fluency, you will feel more and more of the excitement and the magic of the truly lived-in body.

EXERCISING IN
AN OFFICE CHAIR

The idea of little groups of exercises to be done while you take a moment or two from a frantic eight hours is not new. In my file I even have a small, undated booklet titled "Exec's-ercises" and published by the Y.M.C.A. Some of the suggestions in it are very worthwhile. For example: pull in your abdomen whenever the telephone rings, hold while speaking but do not hold your breath; or spend a day not using your arms whenever you stand up or sit down. The amusing cartoon figure is that of a much older-looking executive than we are accustomed to seeing today, indicating key men have improved their breed by heeding this and other good advice.

(If you ever have watched a silent movie or one of the early talking pictures, you must have noticed this social phenomenon: The poor young man struggling to make his way in the world was always thin; his opposite number, the captain of industry, had the mustache of a graying walrus and lumbered about like one, what with his portly front and all. The situation is now entirely re-

---

versed. Most tycoons are muscle-taut and trained down like jocks. The poor, on a diet of TV and fast junk foods, are overweight.)

Here is some updated advice for men and women, executive or otherwise.

1   STRETCH TO CEILING

BENEFIT: To stretch upper torso.

a Sit erect, feet hips' width apart. Breathe deeply as you raise right arm and stretch toward ceiling. Alternate stretch with left arm.

b Perform 5 times, each side.

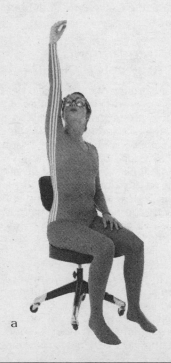

a

2   SHAKE TO FLOOR

BENEFIT: To increase circulation in brain, and relieve stress in back muscles.

a Sit erect, feet wide apart. Stretch arms parallel above head, as you inhale.

b Exhale as you drop torso forward, relaxing arms and head. Hands dangle on floor. Hold for count of 5.

c Inhale as you return to sitting position.

d Perform 5 times.

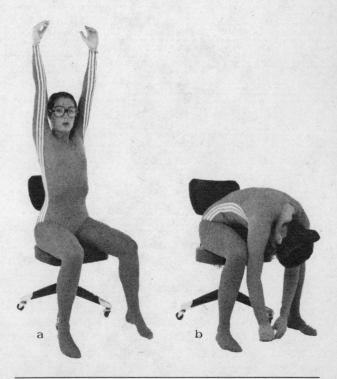

3   WIGGLE

BENEFIT: To stimulate intestinal action and to tone stomach.

a Sit erect with feet together, hands clasped behind head. Breathe normally as you

b Lift right hip and move it forward. Next, inch forward with left hip. Continue to alternate hip movements till you have wiggled to the front edge of your chair. Then wiggle backward to starting position.

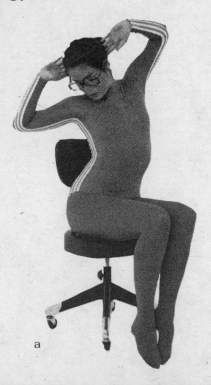

a

4   CRISSCROSS

BENEFIT: To tone abdomen and waistline.

a   Same starting position as above. Inhale.

b   Lift right knee to chest while you twist to
    touch left elbow to raised knee.

c   Exhale, and drop right leg, returning to
    original position.

d   Alternate with left knee and right elbow.
    Perform 5 times, each side.

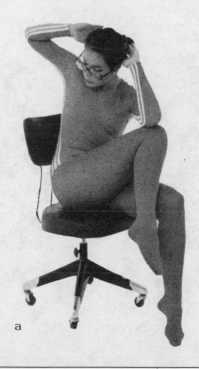

a

5   KNEE HUGS

BENEFIT: To mobilize knee and hip joints after long hours of sitting.

a   Sit erect, with feet about six inches apart. Inhale.

b   Exhale as you clasp hands below your left knee, literally picking up your knee and lifting it to your chest. Hug it close.

c   Exhale and lower your left leg to floor as you continue to control descent with clasped hands.

d   Reverse. Perform 5 times, each side.

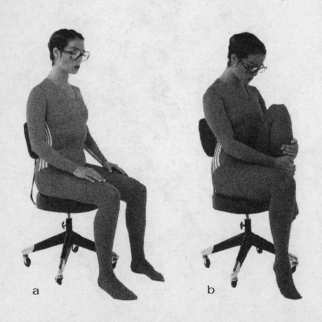

a   b

6 BODY LIFT

BENEFIT: To strengthen arms and abdomen.

a Grasp chair so you surely will be well balanced. Inhale, and pull up legs, feet together.

b Lift body off chair, still keeping knees together, as you conclude inhale breath. Hold for count of 3.

c Exhale, and drop back into sitting position.

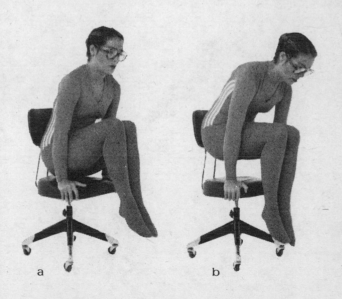

a   b

7   TUCK AND EXTEND

BENEFIT: To firm flabby abdominal muscles.

a Sit erect, legs together. Inhale.

b Exhale as, grasping chair seat, you slowly
   pull knees toward chest and hold for count of
   3.

c Exhale as you extend and straighten both
   legs, keeping knees tight as you drop legs till
   feet touch floor.

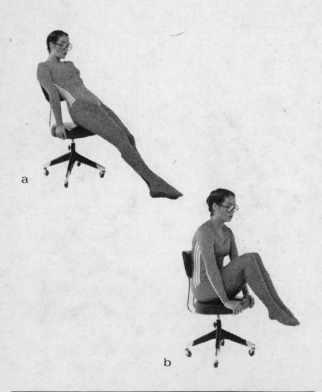

a

b

8 WAIST BENDS

BENEFIT: To stretch waistline muscles, firm upper arms.

a Sit erect, feet hips' width apart. Inhale as you extend arms to your sides, at shoulder level, making right angles to body.

b Keeping elbows straight, bend left arm to left side till fingers of your left hand brush floor.

c Reverse. Perform 5 times, each side.

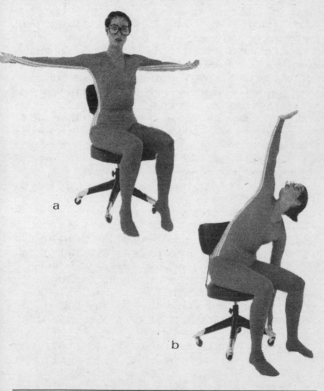

SIX EXERCISE DOS

Remember these six prudent rules for your daily exercise:

1. DO SET ASIDE A DEFINITE TIME DAILY, MONDAY THROUGH FRIDAY. Remember, you can't store the benefits of regular exercise. If you become fit and then cut back to exercising only once a week, you will automatically drop halfway back to your original unconditioned level before ten weeks have passed. And, if you stop completely, within five weeks you'll lose all your gains.

Remember the value of locked-in exercise time. When the children were small, I wore my jogging suit when I drove them to school and headed for the park immediately afterward.

Now I make a firm practice of whipping through the front door at 7:30 A.M., rain or shine.

2. WARM UP SLOWLY. In any exercise session, provide yourself with a few minutes of warm-ups and stretch-outs. Remember how you once warmed up your car for several minutes before you drove off, to make sure the oil lubricated all the parts? A proper warm-up helps ward off injuries by allowing the synovial fluid to lubricate each joint. Do some systematic and moderate bending and stretching.

3. BE SURE YOUR BACK IS READY, TOO. If ever you have been plagued by lower-back pain, do begin with the special back conditioners and strengtheners (page 174).

4. INCREASE YOUR LEVEL OF EXERTION. Recognize that your respiratory/circulatory system is pleading with you daily to pay your dues to your heart by sustained exercise of at least twenty minutes' duration. Afterward, if you so desire, you can zero in on movements for reshaping, slimming down, building up, and otherwise sculpting your ideal form. (See Body Talk, page 160)

5. As your fitness level increases and the urge to do more becomes irresistible, alternate mat exercises with

jumping rope. There are few exercises more timesaving and more satisfying.

6. COOL DOWN SLOWLY. The body, and the heart especially, will protest as much about abrupt, brutal transitions at the end of an exercise period as at the beginning. Stopping suddenly when you have been working out vigorously is just not sensible. Think of the runners in the Olympics, or the horses at the races. They continue to run even after they have ended the race, until their breathing has slowed to a normal rate. Also, it is unwise to conclude any workout with mat exercises that have you down on the floor—get on your feet for the finale!

YOU OWE YOURSELF
A GOOD BILL OF HEALTH

You may wish to know the general level of your heart and circulatory health. And if you're over forty or have any family history of heart dysfunction, I beg you to consult your physician for advice before you take on any rigorous exercise program.

In this regard, a great guide and one I recommend to all Golden Door guests is *Beyond Diet—Exercise Your Way to Fitness and Heart Health* by Dr. Lenore R. Zohman. Developed in conjunction with the American Heart Association and the President's Council on Physical Fitness and Sports, this report may be obtained by sending ten cents for each copy to Consumer Service, Best Foods, A Division of CPC International, Inc., RFD 2, Box 373, Coventry, Conn. 06238.

THREE BASIC
EXERCISE DON'TS

1. DON'T HURRY YOUR BODY. Imagine that you're a gardener. Like a plant, your body is a living organism with certain natural cycles which simply cannot be speeded up. A seed takes its own time about germinat-

ing and growing while you provide the best possible environment and tender care (which includes one irreplaceable ingredient: patience).

2. DON'T BE CONNED BY MOTOR-DRIVEN MACHINERY. When the Golden Door opened in 1959 its gym was agleam with expensive chrome muscle-toners, rollers, and other electric gadgets. I soon threw all these out. Motorized gadgets perpetuate the idle dream that somehow you can have your exercise done for you. Not so. Only you can make your heart pump as strongly as it wants to and should. Physical fitness is something you must get for yourself. And why not, when you are the primary beneficiary?

3. DON'T EXERCISE WHILE HATING IT. Suppose a friend has suffered an illness causing you to fear for your own level of health. Well, that's not a valid reason to start exercising. Negative motivations won't last. Besides, if you exercise with inner tension, rigidity, or anger, every movement becomes tiring. That's because you're working against your total self instead of for yourself.

ELEVEN ABSOLUTE
EXERCISE TABOOS

1. Do not overdo.

2. Do not use isometric-type exercises exclusively. When you do isometric exercises, the blood vessels are contracted by extreme squeezing, inhibiting the flow of blood instead of expanding it. It is only through exercises that aid the flow of blood through the heart and large skeletal muscles that significantly improved cardiovascular fitness is achieved.

3. Do not begin fast-action movement before fully stretching out and warming up.

4. Do not execute *full* deep knee bends if you are unused to them or unused to exercise generally. Until you achieve much flexibility and are proof against kneecap trouble, make it a rule that hips should never be brought lower than the knees.

5. Do not perform hyperextension of the back (backward and forward movements of the torso) without flexing the knee). For instance, keep your knees bent when doing sit-ups.

6. Do not bounce tightly on taut ligaments as you stretch them. (A loose, rhythmic action, however, is great because it is a muscular action.)

7. Never bounce on a stretched tendon; a sustained stretch of a tendon is best.

8. Avoid excessive repetition (overworking a muscle by doing the same exercise or similar ones over and over). Exercise must flow from one movement into another, from head to foot or vice versa. If you remember that the entire body requires movement, you will not overdo on any one body part.

9. Do not lie on your back and lift straight legs without also raising your head, or without bending your knees as you lift your legs.

10. Don't conclude an exercise without a moving cool-down period—one which allows your pulse to return to its normal rate.

11. Don't forget to breathe. This may sound foolish. But I have seen many, many people hold their breath while doing strenuous exercise. Don't perform any exercise without matching it to the normal breathing movements of the lungs. Generally, you should be directed to breathe in when you move upward and to breathe out when you move downward. An exception is when your body is being greatly contracted during an upward movement—that's when you must think of yourself as a concertina and let your inhalation give way to exhalation. And some experts believe that you should exhale during an exercise which puts you in pelvic tilt, since at such a time your abdominal muscles are contracted.

Excessive fast, deep breathing can be as risky as breath-holding. Hyperventilation could make you dizzy or even faint.

THE LOWDOWN
ON YOUR LOWER BACK

It's apparent that a goodly number of these rules are designed to protect the lower back of the middle-aged adult, and with excellent reason. Because of lower-back problems, over $1.2 billion is paid out annually by business and industry in workmen's compensation (but seldom because of incorrect exercising, since most of the victims of whom we speak made the error of taking no exercise at all—see page 20.

You can find the basic rules of back care and exercise in *Care of the Back,* a twenty-four-page pamphlet published by J. B. Lippincott; you can pick up the booklet in most orthopedists' offices.

POOL EXERCISING

As far as I know, Rancho La Puerta and the Golden Door were the first major resorts to rely on water exercises and on water volleyball—both superior forms of exercise, since you always are working against the resistance of the water. You'll know how popular they are if ever you come within a half-block of one of these classes and hear the boisterous, happy noise of the participants.

Swimming and water exercises are considered the most effective exercise for two reasons: 1) they provide a workout for the cardiovascular/respiratory system; and 2) any movement underwater, because of the resistance of the water, will build up the skeletal muscles faster than the same movement done in air.

If you have access to any pool, outdoor or indoor, take advantage of it. Many towns in this country have a pool available for public use; if there is one near you, I can't urge you enough to make it a regular stop.

Don't forget that pool exercises, like every other important exercise activity, require a warm-up period. You can supplement our water exercises by requesting the booklet "Aqua Dynamics" from the President's Council on Physical Fitness and Sports, Washington, D.C. 20201.

GOLDEN DOOR POOL EXERCISES

---

1 JUMPING JACK COSSACK

BENEFIT: Inner and outer thighs.

POSITION: Facing wall of pool. Hands in front of you, grasping pool coping; feet together.

Perform three small jumps in place. On fourth jump, go quite high, splitting legs apart sideways, then landing with feet together. This is a five-beat rhythm: Jump (*slow*), jump (*slow*), jump (*slow*), open (*quick*), close (*quick*).

VARIATION: As you split legs apart on count number four, right leg goes forward and left leg goes back (instead of sideways). Alternate.

VARIATION: When you have perfected the first two versions, then do without the aid of the pool's coping. Instead, stand in the middle of the pool and fold arms Cossack-style as you follow the above directions.

Begin with a set of four each and increase to eight.

---

2 WATER SNAKE DANCE

BENEFIT: Waist and arms.

POSITION: Facing wall of pool at arm's length; elbows straight and hands grasping pool coping; feet together (make sure heels are on bottom of pool). Throughout movement your body remains parallel to wall.

Make four full rotations to right side, four to left: You must avoid twisting torso from side to side as you rotate your hips in a circle. Continue with three full rotations to right, three to left; two to right, two to left; one rotation to right, one to left—by this time, you're really feeling the resistance of the water.

---

3   WALL TO WALL

BENEFIT: The entire body.

POSITION: Standing, facing wall of pool, feet together. Hands holding onto coping, which is arm's length away.

Raise right leg to right side, touching toes to pool wall as you keep right knee straight. As you lean your torso forward, still keeping knee straight and leg high, swing this right leg around in back of you and continue it around in back till your toes touch pool wall on the other side. Bring right leg back to right wall, still keeping the leg as high as possible— as if you were erasing the previous right-to-left movement.

Four times, then reverse and use left leg.

4   WRITING IN WATER

BENEFIT: Waist, hips, backs of thighs, tummy.

POSITION: Back to wall of pool, arms extended at sides, at shoulder level, and resting on pool coping. Right foot, toes pointed, is on bottom of pool in front of you; right knee is straight.

With an imaginary piece of chalk between your right toes, and keeping right knee straight, pretend there is a blackboard sitting in the pool before you, and draw a "V" by raising right leg high toward right side, returning right foot to bottom and then immediately raising right leg toward the left, where it forms a 45-degree angle against your body. Return to starting position.

Alternate with left leg.

VARIATION: Draw a "W" by raising right leg toward

right side, returning right foot to starting position, raising right leg in front of you, returning right foot to bottom of pool in front of left foot, raising right leg to left side. Return to starting position.

Alternate with left leg.

VARIATION: Draw a figure "8." Alternate with left leg.

---

5 CUT THE WATER

BENEFIT: Stomach, arms, legs.

POSITION: Left side is toward wall of pool. Right arm, elbow bent, is crossed over in front of you and hand grasps pool coping. Palm of left hand is pressed against the pool wall, about six inches below right hand; left elbow straight.

Stretch body to its fullest extension, toward center of pool, just as though you were lying on your left side. Scissor legs forward and back, keeping knees straight; perform scissors motion slowly and continue to stretch to fullest extension.

Do ten times. Then roll over to right side, reverse hand position, and repeat all.

---

6 HEAVE HO

BENEFIT: Stomach, backs of thighs, and buttocks.

POSITION: Left side toward wall of pool, left hand grasping pool coping; right leg extended forward at hip height with straight knee, and parallel to water surface; right arm extended back with straight elbow.

Lean your body as far backward as possible. Then bring right arm and right leg down into the water; lean forward as you stretch the right arm forward

---

and the right leg back. (Your knees and elbows remain straight.)

Keep repeating, with a rocking motion of the torso, ten times. Alternate to right side.

---

7 WAISTLINE WIGWAG

BENEFIT: Arms, bust, thighs, waist.

POSITION: Standing in center of pool, feet wide apart, knees bent, back straight. Arms straight out at sides, at right angles to body. Be certain your shoulders and arms are underwater.

Twist upper torso to right side, making sure arms keep their position and do not move either forward or back. Twist torso back to center position and then twist torso to left.

Repeat twenty times.

VARIATION: For upper back and midriff. Back, feet, and legs in same position; hands clasped in front of body; arms outstretched with straight elbows. Arms and shoulders are underwater.

Pivot upper torso from side to side, making sure arms keep their position and do not move either forward or back.

VARIATION: For arms and back of waist. Feet position same. Shoulders and arms underwater. Knees straight. Bending slightly forward from waist, lower your arms and practice golf swings underwater.

VARIATION: For back of arms, pectorals. In golf-swing position, bent over with clasped hands and straight knees, contract your stomach muscles as you unclasp your hands and bring them to the top of the water. Return to starting position, and clasp hands again.

Note: Repeat all variations twenty times.

---

8   BALINESE WATER DANCE

BENEFIT: Waist and arms.

POSITION: Walking position. Shoulders and arms must be underwater. Right arm is outstretched at side, at right angle to body, elbow straight. Left arm, elbow bent, crosses over body with hand pointing toward right. Left arm is held below right arm.

Take your walk across width of pool where water is chest high. Take each step by crossing the stepping foot over in front of opposite foot, so you move from side to side as well as forward.

As you first step forward with your right foot, swing both arms to opposite side—left arm with straight elbow and right arm with bent elbow; both will point toward left after you have swung them through water.

Continue in this way—each time you place one foot in front of the other, swing both arms to the side opposite the stepping foot.

VARIATION: For waist and arms. As soon as you have perfected this, try to do it while backing up.

WEIGHT TRAINING AND SOME EXERCISE ON THE LIGHTER SIDE

If weight training is new to you, don't be put off by the notion that you will have to lift one of those big cumbersome weights and, if you are female, that to do so will induce unsightly muscle bulges. Lady hormones will protect you from the latter. And big barbells are being supplanted by those neat little ankle and wrist weights. Consider purchasing some if, as you normalize your own weight, you see the necessity for concentrating upon certain contours and muscle groups—particularly upon flabby inner thighs, sagging upper arms, and fatty pads at the shoulders.

Begin by snapping on the smallest-size ankle and wrist weights obtainable and then performing your regular exercises, at first very slowly. Later you may wish to experiment with slightly heavier snap-ons.

No less than Colonel James L. Anderson, head of West Point's physical education department, told the Los Angeles *Times:*

> Every woman should overcome her fears and prejudices about weight training. Weight lifting is an efficient way to improve your performance in sports, whether your game is golf, tennis, or swimming. . . .
>
> At West Point . . . we placed a group of 20 high-school women in an intensive weight-training program for eight weeks. All increased their strength substantially but not one developed anything that could be remotely described as bulky muscles.

BREATHE EASY

You're told never to hold your breath while exercising. But I must admonish you never, never to hold your breath while lifting weights. The exertion may make you want to do so but you must concentrate on normal breathing and breathe through the whole process while you lift. Otherwise, you risk a sudden and dangerous elevation in blood pressure.

IT'S ANYBODY'S BALL GAME

Now that women have been accepted in nearly every sport and consequently have the advantage of good professional trainers, I doubt if they have anything to fear from any kind of athletic conditioning. I realized this when, only this spring, I emceed the first annual Women in Athletics awards at California State University, San Diego. These feminine champions didn't look like the cross section of a typical phys-ed class of a few years back. They were simply the most beautiful group of women I had ever seen.

DESIGN FOR LIVING

Don't neglect cycling. A weekend cycling club is family fun. Some lucky people can cycle to work. Consider keeping your bike at the office. A twenty-minute spin can be a more satisfying tension break than the finest lunch.

This very week discover folk dancing; it's wonderful for "family togetherness." Join a group or start up one with your closest friends. When exercise becomes part of your life-style as sports participation and recreation, it is always the most joyous. Of course, don't neglect ski and hiking clubs. Sierra Club members are always super-fit. Consider your friends, and pick people to share recreational activities rather than cocktail parties.

If you feel the need for a complete body redesign, you may want to consult a recommended gym body conditioner. Just be sure your expert does not require you to work out with motorized equipment. Remember, you should provide the energy to operate the equipment. I am keen on Nautilus and Universal-type gyms; we use the latter at the Golden Door.

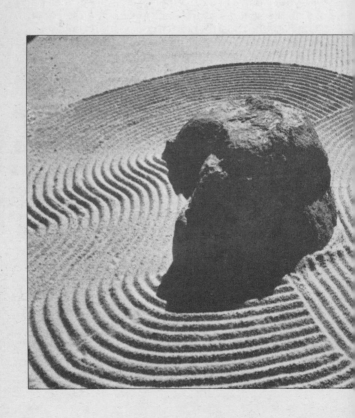

CHAPTER V

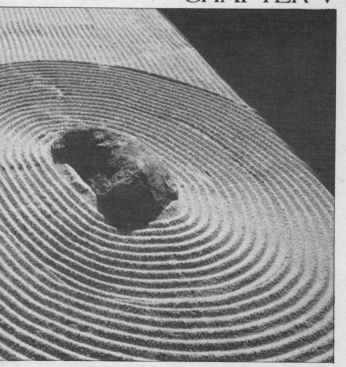

THE JOY
OF JOGGING

> Physiologists used to say that
> good performance resulted from
> being serious, from really pouring it on.
> We're positive now that the time you really
> do something best is when you are
> relaxed and let go of excess tension.
>
> —Laurence Morehouse, Ph.D.,
> professor of kinesiology at UCLA and
> author of *Maximum Performance*

This quote is the fittest description I know for the attitude with which you should approach the easiest and surest road to fitness: the jogger's track or the runner's course. Choose a program and enter in as if it's fun. Soon it will be—fun, and much more.

Ask any runner. You'll be told that the fountain of youth is just half a mile down yonder, that Shangri-la is a few blocks up the street, and the bluebird of happiness which little Mytyl and Tyltyl so earnestly sought is no farther away than the nearest corner.

The other side of the rainbow, you'll learn, is a jogging track.

The phenomenon is worldwide. When in Paris in

1977 (as a member of the President's Council on Physical Fitness and Sports, I was one of two U.S. delegates to the International Conference on Fitness held in the UNESCO palace), one dawn I couldn't help sleepily romanticizing about the clop-clop of carriages I thought I heard in the streets . . . and then I realized that the sound coming through my hotel window was a different sort of clop-clop, made not by nineteenth-century horses but by late-twentieth-century suited-up runners.

THE WORLD AT YOUR FEET

I think jogging has become so popular because the world seems beyond our control, and our government sometimes out of control. We have so many family frustrations. And here is physical effort which will result in something non-frustrating and totally predictable: fitness. Running is the victory of the individual over himself and the world.

We could communicate with the world when it seemed less vast. But now we can no longer think in terms of satisfactory global communication. We have to go back to the individual.

Dr. George A. Sheehan, philosopher laureate of the jogging revolution, puts it this way: "Success rests with having the courage and endurance and, above all, the will to become the person you are, however peculiar that may be. Then you will be able to say, 'I have found my hero and he is me.' "

WHY THE JOGGER'S CUP
RUNNETH OVER

Psychiatrists praise jogging programs for alleviating severe depression in some severely troubled patients.

A vice-principal at a Navajo reservation high school in Arizona spoke for hundreds of thousands of runners everywhere when he explained, "Say you come from work, and you're dead tired. The most logical thing

seems to be to have a beer and take a nap or something. But if you go out and take a run, say seven or eight
miles, *that's like living another day.''*

Mary Healy and Pat Smythe, experts who prepared
the beginner's jogging schedule on page 194, itemize
these specific benefits which all joggers may expect:

1. Nice, firm muscles in legs, arms, back, and
   stomach; less fat overall.
2. Reduction of tension and anxiety.
3. Improved digestion; relief from constipation.
4. Sounder, more restful sleep.
5. Increased self-confidence and self-esteem,
   which can affect all facets of your life.
6. More energy for the rest of your day.
7. More effiicient cardiovascular system.
8. Clearer complexion, better skin tone.
9. Easier weight loss if you're dieting.

RIGHT ON TRACK

A number of these facets bobbed up in a provocative
Baylor College of Medicine report on the testing of personality traits of 48 healthy middle-aged runners. G.
Harley Hartung, Ph.D., commented on test results:
"Most people who become addicted to regular exercise
experience these positive changes—a gain in self-
awareness, in imaginativeness. There's a good chance
they become less neurotic. . . . A regular run won't give
you more brains, that is, but it may help you to use the
brains you've got.''

For me, jogging has been a head trip of another sort.
I'm the so-called picky-perfectionist migraine type.
(See what I'm doing this very moment, revising and
polishing this book, which had been so widely accepted in its original edition. But, no, I had to improve
it, and not because my life is otherwise problemless.
Besides running two resorts, I have increased my responsibility to my community and have just become
immersed in the most crucial and urgent fund-raising
drive I've ever undertaken.) The year I spent as an early

biofeedback guinea pig taught me to control my migraines, to feel one approach and then through concentration to think of it as going away. But running has done even more for me. To the migraine, I am now unapproachable. I seem to have outdistanced migraines, even through the very trying period of a divorce.

HOW TO MAKE IT DOWN
THE HOME STRETCH

Today, at age fifty-seven, I run at least a mile each day, then walk three miles. As a result, I found during the last holidays that I was able to cross-country ski longer and farther than even when I was much, much younger. In fact, I could almost keep up with my children, who are in their twenties.

Each day, before leaving the house, I go through some of the Pre-Anything Exercises (page 110), which handily combine both stretching and a jogging warmup. Then I'm off to jog. Speed isn't important. What counts is moving faster, farther, and for a longer length of time than you customarily do. I still am happiest with doing a full hour upon arising. Then my noon and twilight exercises become a bonus.

Sometimes I still like to alternate with the beginner's run/walk. It's really like a race walk, very feminine-looking—reminiscent in a way of the steps of the coolies whose skirts were so tight they could scarcely move. Race walking has a different pace, a bit of bounce to the ounce. It's very light and effortless.

Then I move on and alternate walk/jog/race walk. Or one day I might walk, next day race walk, next day jog. As I move, I make a point of feeling tall. This puts one's organs in better position.

APRÈS JOG:
IT'S COOL TO COOL DOWN

Regular running made me understand something that used to puzzle me when I was a child watching Fox

---

Movietone newsreels. Why, I used to wonder, did champion runners continue making those long strides minutes after they had broken the ribbon? Of course it's clear to me now that one must keep running, more slowly, till one's breath is under control. It's the cooldown, as important in running or jogging as in any other exercise session.

NEW LIGHT ON YOUR
OLD NEIGHBORHOOD

No, I've never entered a marathon. But if my jog/run accomplishments aren't impressive, my environment certainly is. Grass and sand are the ideal jogging surfaces, and near my home are miles of beaches and one of the world's most glorious parks. My morning jog has taken me to parts of the huge park and through unfamiliar streets I otherwise wouldn't explore. A new appreciation of the out-of-doors is one of the most lush fringe benefits of the jogger. There are sections of your town you've probably never seen, except perhaps from an automobile. Get out and discover for yourself. Be Columbus. Be Audubon.

School grounds, the perimeter of a golf course—there are many desirable and appropriate places to jog. Even the pavement of the city street will do. Studies show that, although joggers in smog and traffic do inhale 40 percent more lead than the slow-moving pedestrian does, they also excrete more. The all-important bottom line comes out in favor of those who really move.

If you run outdoors at dusk or after dark, do take the precaution of wearing light-colored clothing.

RUNNING COMMENTARY

As explained in the beginner's chart, you should always be able to chat or hum while running. If you're too breathless to do so, you're pushing too hard. Try to run relaxed and loose, tensing only the essential muscles. Those muscles not in use should flow along with your general movement. Listen to your breath. Loosen your focus. Try to loosen your consciousness as well (in time, this will happen of itself). Particularly avoid trying to concentrate too hard on counting laps. Don't worry too much about style.

LET ME
SMOOTH YOUR WAY

There are, however, certain pitfalls you must avoid. Don't move in fits and starts. Take care that your back is straight and your head is up; to bend forward will bring on a backache. Bracing yourself with a stiff military posture will have a similar bad effect. And over-striding can strain a hamstring muscle.

Your feet should not be ahead of you or behind you. But don't watch them. Beware of fatigue. If you overdo, you may not be conscious that your gait is changing and that you're jamming your feet down in a way that doesn't absorb the shock that can go right to your knee muscles.

Even if you feel no pain, always stop running when fatigue strikes. And heed this warning above all: Never run on your toes (that's for sprinters).

YOUR JOG TOGS

La Jolla, California, has a new boutique called the Running Shop, and such stores are becoming common elsewhere. I like the commitment that seems to be a natural concomitant of one of those neat jogging suits that zip up the side, but you can get by with soft cotton shorts, cut-off jeans, whatever. Forget the rubberized sauna suits, particularly in hot weather. They are extremely hot and uncomfortable, even dangerous. The weight loss they induce is only water, quickly replaced.

Some people run in street clothes, but here women should be wary of the layered look—running in too many layers of sweat-soaked clothes can drag you down.

YOUR FEET FIRST

The one necessary expenditure is for a nifty pair of jogging shoes. Ask for road-running flats. Good ones cost $20–35. They should be of leather or nylon, with at least one-half inch of cushioning in the sole. They're much better for your feet than sneakers or deck shoes, and you'll know when you have slipped into the proper pair. They'll feel delightful. Adidas, Brooks, New Balance, Nike, Puma, Tiger, all make excellent shoes in a variety of styles. Such chains as Sears and J. C. Penney are finally coming out with fair imitations for under $20. You'll be able to identify a bargain once you know what features to look for.

Remember, each time you lace up your running shoes, that you are making a powerful self-assertion, a statement of will, autonomy, independence, and self-control. The shoes too are a talismanic commitment, symbolic of your new vision of yourself.

RUNNING TITLES

There are so many informative books to tell you much more than I possibly can condense into this chapter. By all means buy a jogging primer, if only the 49¢ Dell *Running, A Complete Guide.* It has a beautiful section on the preparatory phase, the conditioning phase, and an excellent conditioning run-progress chart. This booklet can be found at most supermarket checkout stands.

The only runner I have personally worked with is Mike Spino. He is one of the new breed making running a life's work. His book, *Running Home,* has a number of inspirational chapters on the meditational effects of running.

Fixx's *Complete Book of Running* is that rarity, a how-to book which is gracefully and compellingly written.

One scarcely can keep up with the spate of magazine titles bearing upon the jogging/running boom. *Runner's World* and *The Jogger* still rank among the best. Look them over.

MERRILY YOU MARATHON

For women who are into running, Dr. Joan Ullyot's *Women's Running* is a fine choice. If you have dreams of running marathons, you'll welcome the dandy sample schedules and chapters on marathon running. (Did you know that it's easier for a woman than a man to become a marathon runner? Here is where our more numerous fat cells and muscle cells work in our favor.)

Medical World News, November 27, 1978, tells us that the New York City Marathon drew 423 men and women between the ages of 50 and 60, plus 41 over 60! More than 500 physicians completed this marathon. And 3,000 physicians belong to the American Medical Joggers Association, which emphasizes marathon running.

The Runner for February, 1979, reveals that, in all, 45 states have set 200 marathons for the coming year.

BUT YOU MUSTN'T
LET YOUR ENTHUSIASM RUN
AWAY WITH YOU

If your family has a history of heart disease, if you have been a heavy smoker, or if there is any other factor in your past which must be weighed carefully, marathons and long-distance running are not for you.

Even if you don't belong in any of these questionable categories, if you're lucky enough to live near a practicing doctor of Sports Medicine, by all means ask his advice about any escalation of simple jogging.

Follow Dr. Gabe B. Mirkin's CBS radio show if you're into marathons or long runs. Don't rely on information from the enthusiast loping behind or in front of you. Pay attention to medical experts like Dr. James P. Knochel, who implores runners to stay out of bright sunshine (it can raise body temperature dangerously) and out of marathons conducted when the thermometer registers 85 and above.

YOU KNOW THAT
GREEN LIGHT
THAT SAYS "WALK"?

If, because of age or potential infirmity, you wash out of marathons and long runs, don't look to this book to let you off the hook. Nor will Uncle Sam. My good friend C. Carson (Casey) Conrad, executive director of the President's Council on Physical Fitness and Health, has announced that the government plans a big advertising push. Specifically, it aims to push 45% of the population (who do no form of exercise) off the overstuffed and out onto pedestrian paths and country lanes.

Cardiologists like S. Arthur Leon of the University of Minnesota assure us that "Without stress testing, brisk walking five days a week for at least an hour would give you the same metabolic benefits as the average jogging program."

The buzz word here is "brisk," and Casey means to lean on it, even if he first has to teach everybody *how* to walk.

His particular concern is for the elderly who "have gone through the work ethic. Very few have participated in athletics, and almost none of the women have. They don't think of exercising—they think it's dangerous.

"We have to give status to walking."

WHAT A COMMON, GARDEN-VARIETY BODY CAN DO

Heart specialist Dr. George A. Sheehan says of his book, *Running and Being,* "What I'm telling people is something they already know but have forgotten. . . . A man in one of these urban-renewal areas once said, 'Every adult in the neighborhood is a dead child.' That's the saddest line I ever heard except the one that says the highest percentage of the TV audience is women over 50, which makes me cry. Because I think they're doing that for failure to see their potential, what the common, garden-variety human body can do."

Essentially, Jim Fixx is saying the same thing when, in *The Complete Book of Running,* he lists the needs shared (but not always understood) by all humankind: "The need for movement; the need for self-assertion; the need for alternations of stress and relaxation; the need for mastery of ourselves; the need to indulge ourselves; the need to play; the need to lose ourselves in something greater than ourselves; the need to meditate; the need to live to our own rhythms." He says it all.

The objective of 25,000,000 joggers is not merely one mile, or two, or three. The goal is beyond fitness. The goal is life itself.

A BEGINNING
RUNNING PROGRAM
FOR WOMEN

Prepared especially for the Golden Door by Mary Healy and Pat Smythe (Women on the Run, Inc.; San Francisco).

GETTING STARTED

If you're 30 or more pounds overweight, or 35 years or older, better that you simply should begin walking 20–30 minutes daily, at least five days a week, before you begin jogging. Vary your walking pace, making it alternately brisk and slow. After two or three weeks (or months—age and fitness are the factors here), you may want to alternate slow jogging with walking. As you feel stronger and more comfortable, increase the amount you jog.

Once you've started jogging, plan to commit at least 20 minutes a day, five days a week. That will be sufficient for good muscle tone, weight control, and cardiovascular fitness. If five days are all that your schedule allows for, *never take off two days in a row.* Some people of course prefer to jog every day of the week because of increased benefits.

YOUR RACING FORM

When jogging, maintain an upright posture, neither leaning forward from your hips nor leaning too far backward. Your hips, being the center of your body's gravity, should be in line with your shoulders. Arms should be carried easily in a relaxed position at your waist. Foot plant should be from heel to toe, as in walking. Avoid running on the balls of your feet, where there is little cushion to absorb shock, placing too much strain on calf muscles and Achilles' tendons.

Breathing should always be through your mouth in order to take in as much oxygen as possible. Breathing should not be labored. Running should be done "with" one's breathing, not "ahead" of it. The test: while running you should be able to hum, sing, talk. This is called running at "conversation pace."

INITIAL JOGGING SCHEDULE
(follow for 4–6 weeks)

Sunday	1 mile, or 15–20 minutes of running
Monday	1 mile, or 15–20 minutes of running
Tuesday	day off
Wednesday	1 mile, or 15–20 minutes of running
Thursday	1 mile, or 15–20 minutes of running
Friday	day off
Saturday	1 mile, or 15–20 minutes of running

INCREASED JOGGING SCHEDULE
(follow for 3 weeks)

Sunday	1½ miles, or 30 minutes* of running
Monday	1½ miles, or 30 minutes of running

*Increasing your mileage beyond a 20–30-minute time segment is a matter of individual choice. For good cardiovascular fitness and enjoyment of its benefits, 20–30 minutes of daily jogging is sufficient, and overrunning does not increase the benefits. There is just so much the body can absorb and after 30 minutes the benefits decrease mile for mile

Tuesday	day off
Wednesday	1½ miles, or 30 minutes of running
Thursday	1½ miles, or 30 minutes of running
Friday	day off
Saturday	1½ miles, or 30 minutes of running

MORE ADVANCED JOGGING SCHEDULE

Carefully assess how you feel in terms of fatigue and overall muscular strength before you continue to add on to your mileage. As strength increases, you might add another half-mile two days a week to bring the total to two miles on those days. Follow these basic principles if you attempt to increase your running program. If, for example, you have worked up to two or three miles daily, and want to go for four or even five miles a day, do so in increments. Run only once or twice a week at the longer distance, building to three or four runs at the new distance as you feel comfortable and your body signals that it is adapting to the new demands.

TIPS FOR RUNNING LIKE A TOP:

1. Plan ahead for the days you'll run and those you'll take off. Suit the time of day to your own schedule and needs.

2. Build in many enjoyable variations to your running routine. Run with a friend, run in new locations, plan a pleasant outing after your run.

3. Some of your muscles probably have been inactive for years. Soreness is commonly experienced in your ankles, shins, knees, calves, and Achilles' tendons. Consistency of exercise will minimize the length of time your soreness will remain with you. So will stretch exercises (see pages 112–45) *before and after* running. Depending upon your condition when you begin your running program, your soreness may be mild or intense. In any case, *the soreness can be "run" through.* Don't procrastinate, don't give up.

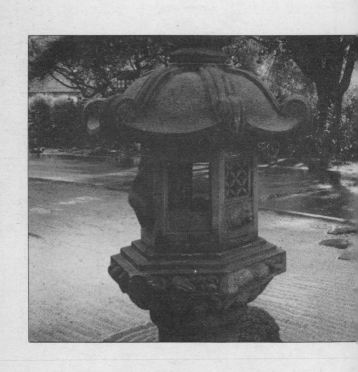

CHAPTER VI

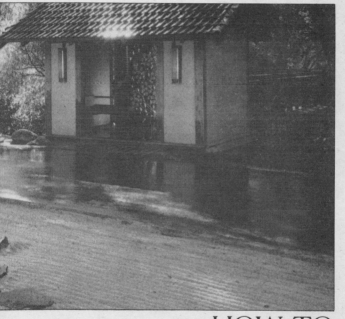

HOW TO
BE HAPPY,
HEALTHFUL,
SELF-FUL

Twenty years ago the Golden Door began with an iconoclastic premise: You do not have to be overweight to have a valid reason to seek our help. You do not even have to be what the French call a woman of a certain age. Turn to the Golden Door simply because you wish to do something for yourself. That we will show you how to be fitter and prettier is almost incidental to the personal growth experience you will undergo. We will show you secrets of removing existing pressures which obscure your better self-understanding and thwart your having a truly joyous life.

This was long before mind trips and getting one's head together and getting in touch with oneself had become standards of the vocabulary. Almost no one was as yet into such experiences. Human potential, as a watchword, was just about to become part of our lexicon. Scarcely anybody practiced meditation. And as yet there was no available body of evidence to indicate that an exercise and resort retreat such as the Golden Door, providing a natural diet and a careful fitness regimen of cardiovascular pulmonary movement plus much opportunity for quiet contemplation and self-examination, could stimulate and free the higher consciousness.

During the Golden Door's first few years, many women who needed and could afford us nevertheless held back simply because they didn't believe they could justify to themselves a full week spent away from work, husband, and family. The whole notion then seemed to them to be tinged with selfishness, the very antithesis of the sweet spirit of self-sacrifice that was supposed to typify the womanly ideal.

This centuries-old prejudice was at length broken down when the more daring ladies who were our early guests amply demonstrated that everything we had promised them could come true: They grew, and consequently they had more to give to those who were closest to them. They could accomplish more on their own behalf, and, to their initial wonderment, still have bountiful energy and enthusiasm for other important commitments as well. Gradually it became accepted that the more one does for one's own mind/body self, the more one is able to contribute in every area touching one's life. This is the very reverse of hedonism.

EVEN THE GREEKS HAD NO WORD FOR THE NEW YOU

Our language hasn't kept pace with this type of enlightenment. Mind-science on the one hand continually instructs us that only loving acceptance of self can make it possible for us to truly love others. Yet the hyphenate *self-love* has overtones of excessive regard for one's own advantage. Our society increasingly sets a new value upon the cultivation of the self. In fact, *Self* is the title of a new Condé Nast magazine, and *Self-Creation* by Dr. George Weinberg was a Book-of-the-Month Club selection. But *"self-esteem"* still carries the connotation of an exaggerated view of one's own importance. And *self-serving* sends no positive messages at all.

In order to express my dearest wish for what you are to become, I need a fresh and unblemished and honorable word. How about:

> self·ful (self·fəl) *adj.,* 1. pertaining to, expressing, or enhancing self-awareness. 2. mindful of personal obligation to the whole self. 3. comfortable and at ease with one's total self. 4. possessing or promulgating self-realization. 5. referring to the most positive characteristics of self-love. 6. pertaining to all self-knowledge and personal development, in the best and highest sense.
>
> See self-fulfillment and self-fruition. —self·fully, adv. self·fulness, n.

WHAT IS YOUR REAL SELF REALLY LIKE?

To be thoroughly, buoyantly, wholesomely self-ful, to be able to resist, overcome, and put behind you whatever detracts from or impinges upon or threatens your invaluable, inimitable self-fulness, you first of all must acknowledge what your self is . . . not alone your physical aspect or the hidden, ineffable you (and if you are naturally shy, I would not for the world have you relinquish all your shyness—after all, it is a trait shared by so many great artists, great thinkers, great scientists). Self is more than the identity who thinks and speaks and acts for you. Part of your self is a psyche that even exceeds mind/body. Self, I would have you agree, is the sum of the you who lives in your mirror and of the you who lives in your mind's eye, of the way you perceive life and react to it, and of all those involuntary processes you merely intuit when you audit your own breathing or heartbeat, or monitor your physical responses via biofeedback.

There are integral parts of your self that you haven't even met yet. My wish is to bring them all together.

Self is the definitive you, and self-fulness the outstanding attribute of the quintessential you.

Blocking this beautiful potential for self-development is that old foe stress, and your attempts to ignore or circumvent it rather than to deal with it.

YOU CAN'T ESCAPE STRESS BUT YOU CAN OUTRUN IT

Stress has always been a concomitant of living, and you cannot and should not ever seal yourself off from either. See stress as growth, challenge, understanding. Sometimes it is even beneficial to intersperse relaxation exercises (pages 73–82) with the recollection of some stressful condition which is troubling you and to give vent to all your feelings about it. But the terrifying fact is that in our age negative stresses are being intensified while at the same time there are fewer and fewer safety valves through which bad stress can be legitimately and safely dispelled.

Because it would be more comforting to believe this is not so, it is a realization which many people try to avoid. As a nation we tend to plunge into life and deny stress—just as we prefer to deny death. Both are allied, and death of course is negative stress's ultimate expression.

What, then, are your options? Whenever you feel pressured, drugs, indulgence in junk food, overeating are very readily available and popular refuges, often paired with sedentary, life-denying recreation. I'm sure you agree in principle that all are bad for you. But since so many people flirt with them in one way or another, you are apt to scoff at the notion that you might be enslaved by any one or combination of them.

So you delay coming to a firm decision about such things. Or you sidestep the fact that such a decision is required of you. And back we come to the Sartrian truth that not to choose is in fact to make a choice.

No one ever actually says, "I am deliberately going to make a lifetime habit of eating junky food, so I can have a junky body"; or, "From this day forward I intend to neglect my body"; or, "I plan to become obese." Also unlikely is "Hereafter I shall drink to excess and go down, down, down!"—an artificial line out of a melo-dramatic old script. But, by your dodging of vital deci-sion-making, these are the end results. They happen little by little as you settle for half-measures and unsatis-factory ways to accommodate your body to the stresses to which it is being subjected.

TO YOUR RESCUE

Although it has been my unhappy duty to warn you against what Dr. Hans Selye terms bad stress—the con-tinuing kind which makes you constantly readjust and readapt—there's good news, too. You can resource-fully turn to powerful natural antidotes. Besides many of the simple and often very pleasing drugless therapies scattered throughout these pages, there is a great trium-virate ready to comfort you: spiritual help through medi-tation or philosophy or religion, together with joyous food and joyous exercise. Fortunately all are compati-ble with one another. And you are already acquainted with my belief that you can best defend yourself from life's slings and arrows by wearing a jogging suit—a veritable suit of armor, I say. Also you are reading daily testimony that jogging can be a first step toward an overwhelming spiritual awakening.

Nor have I run out of silver linings for you. I do side with the experts who agree that when you finally let yourself admit what traps, what ruts, what potentially dangerous reactions you may have been driven to by stress and its relentless assaults, you are at last putting yourself in a position to cope with them.

THE SADDEST
STATISTICS OF ALL

To read you must have light. Only when the sun is shining can you clearly see the peaks and the valleys of your life.

I view life like a mountain range. We begin at the very bottom, a few low hills and gentle dips. As we climb, we develop expertise and we proceed from hill to hill, mountain to mountain peak, searching out the ridges for easier climbing. We avoid the gullies and chasms whenever possible, but here and there we must descend to find the better path. There is always some indecision—which way to go—and often the peak that looks the easiest has a hidden gully, so we turn back to start over again.

Picture yourself as an early explorer, setting landmarks of happy achievement. Each peak reached is a new celebration. But do not try to conceive a happy life as just sitting on any peak, no matter how high it is, for the world will move forward and eventually you will be left behind—alone.

TAKING AN UPPER
IS A DOWNER

The real dangers of drugs of all kinds, as I see them, is that they cause a giant cloud to creep over the life of the climber, a dark shadow that makes it impossible to perceive both the peaks and the valleys, that makes indecision a way of life and renders us impotent.

The *American Journal of Psychiatry* reported a survey by Thomas Craig and Pearl Van Natta in which a community in western Maryland was studied. The "startling findings": within the previous forty-eight hours, more than sixty percent of the 1,059 women and nearly forty-two percent of the 771 men interviewed had taken one or more drugs. Many were resorting to valium, which may worsen depression. When depression is recognized at all, the article said, it is being treated with tranquilizers that at best offer nothing but symptomatic

---

relief, "and, at worst, may intensify the distress they are intended to treat."

The survey revealed that drug usage increased with age. Among those over sixty-five, more than twenty-seven percent of the women and twenty-two percent of the men had taken three or more drugs in the previous forty-eight hours. This survey could have been made in your community, for Washington County, Maryland, is typical of Middle America.

Anxious . . . unhappy . . . lonely . . . depressed . . . all are words which describe the same condition: disease (dis-ease—lack of ease).

FACING UP TO
YOUR MIND/BODY

Let stress problems be your impetus for shaping yourself into the message-receptive, self-ful state into which the Golden Door molds its guests, and then prepare to assume control of your own life. If you have been panicked into drug or alcohol dependency, by all means seek help. Undergo detoxification first. Then unfathom what your mind/body has been trying to tell you, by receiving professional help on a regular appointment basis. Help the professional by making proper exercise and nutrition part of your treatment.

Stress understood can become growth. The decision is your own.

FOR THE WOMAN IN A RUT:
CLIMB OUT OF IT WITH YOUR
OWN TIME-MOTION STUDY

Earlier I wrote that well over half the Golden Door's guests are working women. This should be no surprise, since 50 percent of all American women work outside the home.

Inasmuch as such a lot of time is spent working, in the home or out, how can we go about doing it twice as well, twice as happily? Is it really possible to accomplish everything in half the time?

Here is a secret which took me years to work out. I delight in sharing it. First, you will have to set aside the first week of every month, for several months, to plumb your depths, measure your peaks, and to read your own cycles. All in full sunlight. If you're feeling very low, postpone till a better week.

HOW TO CHART
YOUR PERSONAL PEAKS
AND VALLEYS

Alternate highs and lows of energy are universal, not only apparent in the physical world about us but also within our own inner universe. Chart it.

To be precise, grade your energy on a scale of A to F. Every hour, daily, for the first week, set an alarm clock. Write out the hour and your energy level.

Then examine your chores. From A to F, group them by intensity of effort they require. I'm sure you see my goal. You're going to write each group of chores on graphs, and match the task to the energy level needed to carry it out.

When you're high on energy, positively exuberant with creativity, obviously that's not the time to wash the kitchen floor or to transcribe the morning's letters.

When you're high and creative, review the problem that has been tugging at you for days, feed your soul a good book or a walk in the park.

Save the piddling chores for the hours when you feel low. That's when you balance the checkbook. Shop for groceries. Return routine phone calls.

Some of my most uncomplicated yet productive hours are spent in my car, driving to and from the Golden Door or Rancho La Puerta. Depending upon my energy level, I may listen to tape recordings of seminars, pick a special symphony, or just tape notes for my grocery list.

Soon you too will find that you have made both your high and low hours productive, efficient, and far more harmonious.

WHAT IS THE QUALITY OF LIFE THAT BEGINS AT FORTY?

So often man in his forties is riding a crest. These are his peak years of effectiveness and attractiveness and of reaping rewards. It is ironic and more than a little unfair that a woman's existence may appear to her to be most meaningless at a time when his is most meaningful.

Whether you are a working mother or house mother, if your children, who so often were your first thought upon awakening and your last before sleep, are about to leave the nest, soon you will be alone, probably for the very first time in your life. No wonder the new stress and self-doubts. "Am I too old, too dependent, too discouraged? Am I helpless?" And then the real fears: "Am I unemployable? Does anyone want me?" Add too the possible crisis of divorce; death of a husband; job loss.

Historically we have overcome far greater traumas. Women are survivors, and now you must take yourself in hand rather than take sedatives or alcohol, which serve only to diminish life rather than enhance it. You will have to begin to assess and assert yourself. Train yourself for the new life phase. School, workshops, group therapy, volunteerism, are a few of the many rungs up the career ladder.

VOLUNTEER WORK: A DRY RUN THAT CAN BE YOUR WELLSPRING

What is your new arena of activity to be—school, career, or volunteer work? I hope you haven't been biased by some of the diatribes against the concept of women as volunteers. There has been a shortsighted attempt to inject the suspicion that the performing of services without pay is somehow demeaning. You can see what nonsense this is when you reflect that our country not only does not subsidize the arts but has virtually abandoned them to the suzerainty of the female sex. Hardly a symphony, community theater, local museum, hospital, or school could exist today if all women volunteers withdrew. Do stop by any candidate's office during a campaign year. Notice that without women volunteers the whole system would dissolve.

Whether your predilections impel you to work for the cause of the arts or with humanity at a more mundane level, to make a beginning in satisfying services is to follow Dr. Selye's instructions to conquer stress by doing something which you enjoy and which others appreciate. And you soon will glory in your newfound abilities, new friends, new points of view.

There also are practical aspects to be considered. If you have never been employed, or if in earlier years you held some dead-end job as a clerk or typist, a volunteer capacity that involves responsibility and decision-making can be ego-building and act as a dry run for a future career. If take-home pay is to be the next rung of your ladder, you will benefit greatly if you can afford the time to try on some volunteer jobs for size. A woman in midlife who heretofore has not worked or has been out of the job market for many years is apt to have no more clear-cut view of the direction her plans should take than has a confused sixteen-year-old when first thumbing through a college catalog.

THE MIDLIFE CRISIS
AND THE THIRD-LIFE CAREER
(Where Do I Go from Here?)

Your early decades confront you with more growth troubles, more difficulties, and deeper problems than you should be encountering later. But if you continue the very same paths, they will only lead you to ever-deeper ruts and ever-higher and more rigid walls. Or you can put an end to it, and say, "I've had enough. I will learn from experience. Hereafter I'll not repeat my mistakes."

Study the values you've been living by. In all probability they were formulated when you were sixteen.

You no longer wear the same clothes, and perhaps not even the same dress size. Why, then, continue in an old-time life-style?

Our parents came from one era. We belong to yet another. We have to free ourselves from some of the false values that society often lays on us.

YOUR TIMES, THEY ARE A-CHANGING

If you will accept change within yourself, the midlife crisis can be the opportunity for your most positive growth. Your hierarchy of needs has evolved. The uncertainties of youth are part of your past. Now is the time for reappraisal.

Since everything is changing so rapidly about you, why not get on top of that change and direct it upward?

This period in your life doesn't differ all that much from your adolescence, which after all you survived. It was then that you first moved from the security of your known world out into the future with all its perils.

But today you can rely on greater self-knowledge and a more objective view of your potential. Plan to live for what is important to you. Discard other people's value systems. Remember that you have limited time to waste.

"YOUTH IS WASTED ON THE YOUNG" (RETOOLING FOR THE THIRD/THIRD)

George Bernard Shaw said it. He knew whereof he spoke. A careful vegetarian and fitness enthusiast before such types became common, he wrote some of his major plays when past eighty, and in fact continued to write until he died, at the age of ninety-four.

A man's or a woman's life can be divided into three thirds: the first, growing up—acquiring the ability to think and to work, to receive education and apprenticeship. Second, work for marriage, children, family life, and physical and emotional confidence (this, of course, includes making money). Third, work for our pleasure—

collaborating to ameliorate all aspects of our cultural and community life.

The third/third of life should be the most pleasing, for we begin at our highest pinnacle of knowledge, experience, ability, and—if we work at it—fitness. Utopia is our goal, and we who have the highest standard of living and human concern must lead the way.

To live fully, the whole of one's life span, a sharp and effective body/mind is a must. One cannot wait until fifty to create the tool of which I speak. Preparation for the third/third is vital—one cannot begin to study the alternates after retirement. Mind/body flexibility is quite easy to maintain but extremely difficult to acquire once lost. An increasing, but yet small, number of businesses offer scholarships for retraining, retooling for the fifty-year-old. That should be one of our major goals, rather than a better pension, for all hands (and minds) are needed to prepare the millennium.

Until that day comes, each of us must survey our own energy reserves, and—if and when they are low—increase the deposits of life-enhancing foods and actions. Hence today, at 57, I allow myself a minimum of exceptions to both my exercise schedule and food plan, for I believe in living for life.

An analogy I use when I lecture to men guests at the Golden Door is to ask them to conjure up a vision of a large tree supported by one tap root and a few weak roots. Such a tree is a man who devotes himself exclusively to his one job, the man we often call the compulsive workaholic. Retirement for such a person is like severing the tap root, and the first wind will blow the tree over. Now, conjure up the long-lived trees in nature, which have roots that extend to and often beyond the diameter of the branches. Even if you sever the tap root, the tree will hold and continue to grow, for many roots carry its nourishment.

My audience quickly sees the analogy to the many-dimensional person each of us must become if we are to thrive in our third age.

DON'T SPRING THE
TRAP OF LONELINESS

Beware of loneliness. It has been termed a massive national problem. Philip E. Slate in his book *The Pursuit of Loneliness* says that American culture as we know it today frustrates three basic human desires: the desire for community, the wish to live in trust and cooperation with others; the desire for engagement, the wish to come to grips with social and interpersonal problems; and the desire for dependence, the wish to share responsibility for the control of one's impulses and the direction of one's life. Loneliness affects all ages, all people, but it is saddest for the elderly. After a certain age the habit of sharing, giving, and receiving is hard to relearn.

That is why the expanded family of bygone days must now be replaced with friends—not one or two, but many. This one for working hours, that one for study hours, another for hugging, another for travel companionship. And what about a partner for tennis? You need to support each other, in times of crisis, and also for increase of joy.

I cannot speak of loneliness without adding a few thoughts about love, which, when truly shared, is more than doubled. Two can grow together and each one thereby increase his or her own power of being. Love is indeed the moving power of life. How wonderful to love another person wholly, and to have that love returned. But if you cannot have the one big love, the many little ones can suffice. Friends, children, nature, your very own self—cultivate them all and add to your joy and your life, year by year.

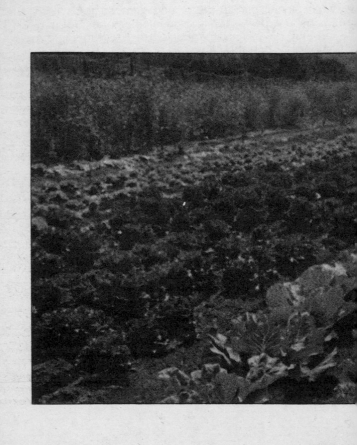

CHAPTER VII

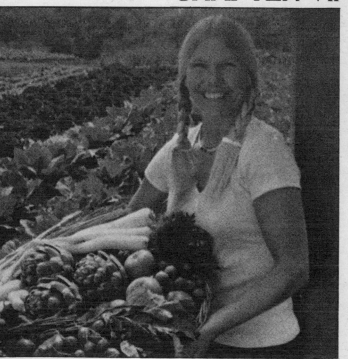

WONDER
WEEKEND

One day in the early 1950s when I was walking along a path at Rancho La Puerta, I thought I recognized someone who avoided me by ducking behind the gym. "Who was that?" I asked one of the staff. "Oh, that's the lady you were so proud of when she left here four months ago. She is very embarrassed and doesn't want you to see her till she has lost the twenty pounds she regained."

If I were to be proud of my life's work, I saw then, it was vital not to conduct a mere "fat farm" where one takes off a few pounds only to put them on again. I wanted to provide a lasting program that would eliminate from my guests' lives the need to play such a sad game. And so—the philosophy of the Golden Door.

The French phrase—*reculer pour mieux sauter*—

comes closest to expressing the essence of the Golden Door: to draw back in order to make a better leap forward. After all that I have said about fitting a program of well-being around your place in the real world, it may seem paradoxical for me now to be advising you to draw back from daily life. But you will have to retreat for a bit so that you may create your own Golden Door.

THE GOLDEN DOOR—
YOUR SOLO HONEYMOON

After her most recent visit, Joan Konner, who has produced so many NBC specials, wrote to thank me for having provided "such a wonderful place for a honeymoon with myself."

"The Golden Door is a heavenly sanctuary," writes Barbara Howar, journalist, television personality, and novelist. She flies out regularly from Washington, D.C.

"I'm so relaxed when I get back," she once confided to *Harper's Bazaar,* "it takes me about six months to start screaming at the children."

Recently she told me, "Everything that happens to me when I leave the Golden Door is wonderful. When I get my stomach flattened and my head straightened, things just seem to come together nicely. All I really need is one more 'pit stop' a year at the Golden Door."

GO CLEAR OUT OF THIS
WORLD SO YOU CAN
FUNCTION BETTER IN IT

Each of us needs sanctuary. I provide one at the Golden Door by permitting a guest to pause and gather herself in a quiet, remote, other-worldly environment.

The first time Rita Bronowski walked into the Golden Door, it was to escape a devastating emptiness following the sudden death of her husband, Dr. Jacob Bronowski, noted mathematician, scientist, and philosopher whose *Ascent of Man* became a highly praised educational-television series and bestselling book. She sought a refuge where she could deal with her emotions before facing unfamiliar responsibilities.

"I left with a deep sense of the Golden Door's power to heal. It was astonishing that the pressure of all the jobs piling upon me—the unanswered mail, bank details, insurance muddles—seemed lifted."

The second time Rita was a guest at the Golden Door, it was for the purpose of being deliberately "shaken by exercise, jolted completely out of old habits, cleansed mentally and in every sense."

Since then, she has begun to edit several volumes of her late husband's lectures. There's still time daily for a brisk hour-long walk that helps her "feel like a million and ready to tackle it all."

HOW I DISCOVERED
MY OWN GOLDEN DOOR

Paradoxical or no, retreating for a serene and solitary weekend has helped me many times to collect my own energies. Since the Golden Door is my business, it can provide no "heavenly sanctuary" for me. Yet there was a time in the late 1950s and early 1960s when I desperately needed a Golden Door-like haven which would give me the time and the perspective to review my life, refill my reservoirs, and make some sense of the future.

I had two very young children and felt tremendously responsible for providing a good life for them, even while I realized I was losing my husband. I knew I would have to be both father and mother.

In addition, I was responsible for running two major health spas. The Golden Door, the second of the two, was just starting on the proverbial shoestring and with all the turmoil attending the birth of any ambitious adventure. My days began at six and ended well past midnight, and every day was a struggle.

I looked at myself and thought, "Well, I can choose to have a nervous breakdown, to get sick, or to do something about it all." I decided to take a long weekend all by myself at a little resort nearby. There was nothing fancy about the place; it was just blessedly quiet.

PACK UP YOUR TROUBLES

Just what I was going to do, I didn't know. Because I was too exhausted to take my usual stacks of work, I threw some clothes into a bag along with a Ray Bradbury science-fiction book and—because I had found it lulling reading—Jean-Paul Sartre's *Being and Nothingness.* My state then was not unlike that of three thoroughly vital and very overcommitted women whom I admire, who at one time sought the Golden Door for the same reason—to escape the pressure of excessive demands. When their physicians had prescribed total rest and suggested the hospital, Shana Alexander, Barbara Howar, and Beverly Sassoon came to the Golden Door instead. There, each found within herself her own strengths. Stress studied is the best precondition to change.

At that time, however, I did not realize I was setting up my own "Lilly tank," my own space for sensory deprivation. I did not know that it also would be my "growth" tank, a refuge where I could think about my life and marshal my strengths.

The first day I did nothing except swim, eat, read science fiction, and gaze into the fire.

The second day I awakened at dawn feeling restless, went for a really long walk, and reached the crest of a small hill just in time for sunrise. So I began my day with a nature high.

After lunching and napping, because I felt good about myself and had nothing else to do, I picked up Sartre and came upon a phrase in *Being and Nothingness* that has given direction to my life: "Freedom is the freedom of choosing but not the freedom of not choosing. *Not to choose is, in fact, to choose not to choose.*"

YOU CAN'T LEAVE YOUR PERSONAL CROSSROADS TILL YOU MAKE A CHOICE

This simple phrase did it. I knew the choice was mine and that I would elect to lead a different sort of life. By the third day I was driving home, singing happily to myself.

Long ago Socrates said, "The life which is unexamined is not worth living." Pogo more recently said, "We have met the enemy and they is us." I know there are dozens of variations, all leading to the same conclusions. But again I'll quote Sartre, who puts things so well: "A free being is one who makes decisions relating to his past in the light of his future and who does not let himself be determined by the present."

From that day forward, I took responsibility for my life.

Rather than trying to avoid stress, I came to think of it as another term for growth. I saw that I must choose how to react to stress.

YOUR GOLDEN DOOR
WONDER WEEKEND

How to be alone creatively? If, physically, you become what you eat, it follows that, mentally, you become what you think. To encounter yourself, you must do as I did that weekend many years ago. First, get away from your daily life. I suggest that you seek a quiet hotel in the country. Just slip into the hinterland. You shouldn't have to drive more than a hundred miles from home. If your destination has paths to walk along, if there's peace and quiet, you've found your place.

For many people, the prospect of being alone for two days is disconcerting. But only by being alone and allowing the tide of communication to ebb can you see clearly to your own depths and recognize your own patterns. You will treasure the moment when you can be as a solitary pebble dropped in a still pool, and the ripples of thought you release are disturbed by no intrusion.

> How can any one of us
> be alone?
> Open a window and

                    life opens for you ocean-wide
                    filling and spilling
                        the playful harmony
                        of being.

I quote from a card my daughter wrote for me as I set out
for a recent series of my own country weekends. I'll be
talking about these presently.

Appreciate the delights of ritual. You've picked out
your retreat and set aside the free time. While you are
packing, consider two elements that will add to the
pleasurable impact of your weekend: ritual and cherish-
ing.

There is a ritual to each aspect of a day at the Golden
Door. People are pacing off to classes in their kimonos
and warm-up suits. All know why they are there, and
are in a meditative state beyond thought. There is a
sense of serenity and order and purpose.

Cultivate that sense of ritual during your weekend. A
simple process like bathing can be turned into a rite.
While you are setting out the soap and shampoo and
scent and an assortment of different-textured towels,
think about the liquid luxury of your bath. Afterward,
cherish the bath itself.

Cherish yourself and your reactions to everything that
gives you comfort and sustenance.

Start deciding while you pack how many ways you
can make the entire weekend a series of rituals. Then
you will have freed your energy for other thoughts.

What things to bring? You will be doing a lot of walking. Good walking shoes and your favorite old clothes
are all you will need. Pack a bathing suit if there is a
place to swim.

Also include whatever recreational pleasure-givers
are sure to loosen and relax you—but no drugs and no
hard liquor. Books are delightful companions. If you are
more aural or tactile, bring along a musical instrument,
or a sketchpad, or needlepoint, or binoculars for bird-
watching—whatever eases you into a peaceful, contemplative state. You must also bring a notebook, a
tape measure, and, finally, your calendar for several

months past; plus five felt-tipped pens of different colors
—black, blue, red, green, and deep lavender. A little
later, I'll explain why. You should always keep a personal and business calendar. Make it as detailed as
possible. You need to become aware of the most precious ingredient of life—your time. The ways in which
you use it will define your life.

THANK GOODNESS
IT'S FRIDAY

Friday evening: Arrive, unpack, settle in. Your experience actually begins at dawn on Saturday.

For the time being, revel in the thought that these
hours are all your own. Relax. Read, have a glass of
wine if you like, and go to sleep early. Set your alarm for
sunrise. That is important. You are going to begin
afresh, and there is nothing more fresh than a newly
created day.

SATURDAY: YOUR VERY
OWN RHYTHM OF LIFE

Saturday at dawn: Walk out just as the earliest rays of
the sun catch the treetops. Stride out briskly, breathing
deeply. Once you feel the warmth of exercise, begin
changing the pace. Look around you. Slow down to
inspect some special tree or flower, then speed up
again until you are breathing strongly and have felt the
warm glow that is followed by cooling sweat. Time to
slow down again. Alternate for forty minutes; then,
back to your room.

8:30 A.M. After cooling off, bathing, and dressing,
you probably will be ready for breakfast. Avoid order-
ing your usual meal. Rather, listen to your body and let
it suggest what to eat. Are you really hungry? Early-
morning exercise affects people differently. Some
come in ravenous, looking for a big farm-style spread.
Others have feasted on oxygen and need only a few
calories and a little protein to sustain their high. Do what-

---

ever feels right but remember that the bigger the break-fast, the smaller the dinner.

9:00 A.M. For about an hour, find refuge in some sheltered nook. Sit and read, sketch, or play a tune—whatever you enjoy. Experience quietness. Don't think back or ahead. This is a nonthinking day, a turning-off day so that tomorrow can turn you on. We need to leave behind the tyranny of the past, and the dominance of the present, if we are to delight in the future.

10:00 A.M. Now, into movement for about an hour. Your surroundings will suggest the activity: a walk, tennis, horseback riding, swimming, whatever the opportunity affords. Perform vigorously, and at a pace that makes you breathe hard and feel tired but not exhausted.

Alternate being active and quiet throughout the entire weekend; in an analogous way, the weekend itself and others like it will be alternatives to your life's busy-ness and tension. Extend the principle of alternation to almost everything you do. Be conscious of your reactions to bright sunlight as opposed to cool shadows, to input from nature in contrast to occasionally shutting off your perceptions of the physical world. Such contrasts keep us alert and elastic.

11:00 A.M. Time for either a swim or a shower. Don't hurry. Start off with the water mildly warm, then shift to very, very hot, then cool down to icy cold. Feel the water, the cleansing, and the baptismal significance. Dry off slowly and languorously, switching between smooth and rough towels.

11:45 A.M. Devote fifteen minutes to enhancing the body awareness induced by your shower or swim. Wearing as little clothing as you can, find some radio music that suits you. Dance slowly, and later quickly, about the room. Of course you are self-conscious. Acknowledge your feelings, but continue. Stretch out each limb. Be a rag doll and rotate your neck. Shrug your shoulders. Tug on your hair. Massage your scalp muscles. All over your body, tighten and relax each muscle group, one at a time.

12:30 P.M. To lunch. Order something simple, low-calorie, and vegetarian. Have a large fresh-fruit salad with some raisins or nuts, or a vegetable salad and cottage cheese. Eat slowly and consciously, with awareness of the food. Use all your senses. What is the taste, the smell, and the textural feeling of the food in your mouth?

2:00 P.M. You've been up since dawn. You might want a nap after luncheon. Or you might prefer a tour of the area, visits to antique or book stores, or a bicycle ride.

Fine-tune your senses. Let your eye be caught by the curious, the offbeat.

4:00 P.M. You might read or walk. There is no sacred schedule. Just stay with the principle of alternative activities. The morning walk, so many hours ago, set you experiencing the day (not thinking it) in a receptive, sensitive way.

7:00 P.M. Dinner. Indulge yourself. Either order a big meal, with a glass of wine and all the trimmings, to reward yourself for a day well spent; or glow with virtue and tuck into another vegetarian feast.

8:30 P.M. Avoid the desensitizing effect of banal TV programs and the late news. Bring out a book, or light some incense and respond to your favorite music.

SWITCH YOUR
MINDSET TO "IDLE"

This is a good time to play your own biofeedback-inspired relaxation game. Think a moment about how you can make it work for you. Imagine a physical reaction which is the diametric opposite of the harsh stresses of modern living. Picture your pulse slowing down; your breath subsiding to slow, slower, deeper; and all the tension oozing out of your fingertips, your toes, your entire body. Step by step, feel the unwinding of tension giving way to peace. Visualize whatever pleases and soothes you: Bands of ultramarine and aquamarine water along a coast silent except for seabirds, jeweled with tide pools perhaps never explored by man; a convent garden replete with heavy-headed rose blossoms and respectful bees, a sundial, and the occasional chiming of a bell; an Arabian Nights oasis enfolding you with the shade of date palms beside the splash of a delicate, deliberate fountain.

There's a normal pattern to relaxation, just as there is to movement. Not half as hard as yoga or meditation, it's an inward ability you can master at will.

Now, the Saturday tides which surged forward during the day have reached time for ebbing. No longer try to focus very clearly on anything. Your sleep should be deep and restorative. Its blessing will renew you for the morning.

AFTER THE
SATURDAY SLOWDOWN;
THE SUNDAY SHOWDOWN

You will have noted, and perhaps with disappointment, that Saturday is a do-nothing, think-nothing day. For the weekend with yourself—to duplicate the special magic of a Golden Door week—you require first the contrast of mindlessness, a time for the pieces to fall apart before you can pick them up and put them together in the way you desire, and thus fashion your life as you wish it to become and to be.

Sunday at dawn: Make this truly the first day of the rest of your life—the day of choices, to be approached with a positive viewpoint. Out you go again for the forty-minute walk that marks the day's beginning. That fresh air, with the high it gives you, is a must for what is to follow.

8:30 A.M. A small breakfast, so you will be alert and sharp.

9:00 A.M. Now you have the whole morning for talking to yourself. Make sure that the you who answers is in a strong and happy mood. If not, skip it. Today is not the day. Negative thoughts and feelings should not be entertained as you set about choosing.

The self-fulfilling prophecy we are planning is the one nature destined you for.

YOUR BODY INVENTORY

Your mind/body is what puts it all together and makes it all come true.

Ready? Off with your clothes. Begin in front of a mirror. Think of yourself as an artist. Judge the aesthetics of your appearance. Check for harmony, proportion, and vitality. What is the message given by your hair, your eyes, your skin, and your posture? What does the picture tell about the inner you?

Is your mind/body blighted by neglect or radiant with loving concern? Never forget that this is the tool with which you will carve your life.

Chart your own country. Write down your weight and your height. Measure your hips, waist, and bust or chest. Use these body statistics as a starting point rather than as a means of comparing yourself to Perfect Person.

Form an idea of how much excess fat/fuel you're carrying; visualize those extra pounds. Take them off with your mind's eye and set them down, *there,* on the table. Heavy, aren't they? Of course they have been slowing you down, both physically and emotionally. Each pound represents more unnecessary work for your heart and lungs. If you are average, you will live into your late seventies. What will your life, physically, be like then? This too is a decision you're making today.

Although appearance tells a lot, even more revealing is your body's response to activity. So you must measure your body's endurance, flexibility, and strength.

YOUR ENDURANCE (THE STEP TEST). Good health is more than skin deep. The endurance that gives you steady, glowing vitality under stress comes from your cardiovascular/respiratory system.

Sit down and relax for a minute or two, then take your pulse (count for thirty seconds and multiply by two). Do it again to check the accuracy of your count. This is your resting heart rate. Write it down.

Next comes a test of your heart's response to physical exertion. The President's Council on Physical Fitness

---

recommends the two-minute Step Test for this purpose. It is not difficult. It informs you how quickly your heart returns to normal after exertion, and is a simple test of circulatory efficiency.

You perform the Step Test by stepping up and down, onto a bench, chair, or step fifteen to seventeen inches high. Here is how the President's Council bulletin describes the Step Test:

> Count One—Place right foot on bench.
> Count Two—Bring left foot alongside right, and stand erect.
> Count Three—Lower right foot to floor.
> Count Four—Lower left foot to floor.
> Repeat the four-count movement thirty times a minute for two minutes, then take your pulse. Write it down. Now rest for two minutes, and again take your pulse. (You can find the pulse by applying middle and index fingers of one hand firmly to the inside wrist of the other hand, on the thumb side.) Record the count.
> Rest again for two minutes and take your pulse, recording it for future comparisons.

As your lifelong fitness program progresses, you will find your heart becomes more efficient. The measure of that efficiency will be a lower pulse rate on the first measurement after stepping, and less of a difference between that and the second measurement. As the difference between the two decreases, you see the approach of fitness. (Take future tests at about the same time of day, and use a bench or chair of the same height.)

Endurance develops slowly. You can, however, make yourself appreciably more flexible in just a few days.

TESTING . . . TESTING

Your flexibility: Stand straight, feet twelve inches apart, arms hanging loosely. Bend forward slowly,

---

knees straight, and try to touch your toes. Do not lunge or strain; stop when you feel pain. Do it again with a tape measure. Write down the distance from your extended fingertips to your toes. If you can't touch your toes now, you should be able to within a very few weeks after starting your stretching and limbering exercises (see Body Awakeners, pages 59–102). Eventually you may be able to touch your toes without flexing your knees. But don't push for this if you are stiff or have a history of back trouble. Very easy does it.

Now test your hips. Hold one arm out in front of you with the palm of your hand about six inches above waist height. Now swing up the leg on that same side, and try to touch your big toe to the hand, keeping your knee straight. You should be able to swing your leg forward above the horizontal. If you're stiff, it's most likely because you haven't been using certain joints, tendons, and ligaments, and partly because of tension in the body. It is a condition that improves quickly as you work on it.

Your strength: Strength in the abdominal area is important, since those muscles directly affect posture. The simplest test for abdominal strength is the sit-up. Lie on your back with your knees comfortably bent and your arms above your head. Sit up. Count the number of times you can do it. Write them down.

Now test your arm power with knee push-ups. Lie on your stomach, hands under your shoulders. Keeping your back straight, use your arms to push yourself up until, with arms extended, your weight rests on your hands and knees. How many can you do? Write down the total.

Finally, the leg muscles: Stand on your toes, back against the wall, arms horizontal in front of you. With your back straight, bend your knees and squat with your buttocks no lower than your knees. Then come back up to a standing position. How many times can you do this? Write down the total.

You now have a sheet of figures for weight, height, hips, waist, and bust; for heart rate at rest, immediately after a Step Test, two minutes after, and four minutes after; for toe touches; for sit-ups, knee push-ups, and squats—and you now have a much more finely tuned sense of your own body than you had an hour ago.

Watch yourself grow younger. Now make a note on your calendar to take another Body Inventory at the end of next month. After that, inventory every three months. As you compare each set of new figures with the old ones, you can watch yourself grow younger. As you begin to watch your results and feel the impact of fitness on your daily life you will be surprised at your behavior modification. Just like Skinner's pigeons, you will be enticed by immediate gratification. You will start—again I quote from Sartre—"to obey nature in order to command it."

YOUR IDENTITY INVENTORY

Now, you need to find out about your most private, honest self. This is not a time for rationalizing or wishful thinking. We have been discussing the technique of communicating with your inmost self. Now you're going to ask that self many questions. You already know all the answers but to communicate them may require a new vocabulary. (One you can acquire readily enough.)

Understanding yourself involves, for the most part, a kind of quiet listening to the mind. It's no accident that most philosophers, inventors, scientists, mathematical geniuses, and great musical composers have been quiet people.

Don't be frightened by what you may hear from within. There's a normal tendency to withdraw from the new and strange; some inner trembling can be expected. Moving toward self-knowledge is like moving from the dark into the light.

The most expeditious way to begin is the way journalists do, by setting down the answers to their standard formula of five questions beginning with the letter "w."

YOU, IN CLOSE-UP

Who are you? Jot simple things like name and address, single or married—anything you think pertinent to a brief physical and psychological description of yourself.

WHERE ARE YOU

Have you a sense of belonging in some one place? Are you rooted or mobile? What paths have you worn across the landscape? Where do you fit in this world?

Are you satisfied with your *where?* Is it the proper way station for the route you wish to travel? Today in some states the number of adult part-time college students exceeds the full-time students of traditional college age. Women in particular have many new opportunities for fulfillment, and all mature Americans should be revising their personal road maps.

A real decline in energy and strength doesn't often set in until after sixty; sometimes not even then. Remember that you're not in a trap unless you yourself are constructing one. When we feel chronic fatigue and depression, sleep poorly or don't eat well, or find ourselves inattentive at work or at the wheel of the car, these are just early-warning signals. You're being put on Red Alert about an approaching crossroads crisis. Consciously choose to use its intrinsic stress as a springboard to a fresh, better, more joyous plateau.

We should always be more dreams ahead than we are dreams behind.

WHY DO YOU DO WHAT YOU DO? What is your commitment? Are you in the right place at the right time for you? Are you convinced that you're doing something of value? A sense that your life should be meaningful is too critical a priority to be ignored.

Abraham Maslow believed that self-actualization— the complete expression of one's potential and feelings —should be everyone's goal. People who have confidence in their own value system and feel they can control what happens to them, good or bad, generally are the happiest.

I'm not expecting you to put in your thumb and pull out the plum of happiness on the first try. Just learn to enjoy the pursuit.

WHAT DO YOU DO AT WORK TIME? This, the first question we put to a stranger, is our way of asking about many other things too. What kind of person are you? What do you believe in? Do you think of yourself as having a job title? What are your patterns of activity? What is your life-style? Your satisfaction with your performance is integral to your pride in yourself. Through work, we handle most of life's anxieties; we gauge our own growth primarily in terms of work.

WHAT DO YOU DO WITH YOUR LEISURE? People who achieve the more-or-less average age of seventy-five years harbor more regret for what they didn't do than for the things they did. If you attain that average age, you'll be looking back upon some twenty years of working and twenty-five years of sleeping. For many people, this is almost involuntary apportionment of their time. It's only the remaining thirty years which they were free to shape and form.

Passing time already has whittled away at some of your total of thirty. You'd better get on with them. All you may have to do is redirect and revise your use of time. To recognize this is prerequisite to all achievement. Meaninglessness is more frightening than death. Challenge attempted is what makes an ego grow powerful and sure.

WHEN FATHER TIME
AND MOTHER NATURE

When is the time factor. It includes your age and your sense of how much future you have. What time is it in your life? Is the dotted line on your life graph curving up or down?

Of all the five questions, that concerning physical and psychological (as opposed to chronological) age is the easiest to assess and influence. A simple change in dietary and living habits can accelerate or decelerate the aging process. I believe you already understand this. Act on this understanding, and you can look, feel, and virtually become younger.

Since it is apt to be more accurate, respond with your first impulse to all of the above self-questions, as well as to the following questionnaire by Lilburn A. Barksdale:

BARKSDALE
SELF-ESTEEM EVALUATION*

Score as follows (each score shows how true OR the amount of time you believe that statement is true for YOU):

0 = not at all true for me

1 = somewhat true OR true only part of the time

2 = fairly true OR true about half of the time

3 = mainly true OR true most of the time

4 = true all the time

Score   Self-Esteem Statements

_____ 1. I don't feel anyone else is better than I am.

_____ 2. I am free of shame, blame, and guilt.

_____ 3. I am a happy, carefree person.

_____ 4. I have no need to *prove* I am as good as or better than others.

_____ 5. I *do not* have a strong need for people to pay attention to me or like what I do.

_____ 6. Losing *does not* upset me or make me feel "less than" others.

_____ 7. I feel warm and friendly toward myself.

_____ 8. I *do not* feel others are better than I am because they can do things better, have more money, or are more popular.

_____ 9. I am at ease with strangers and make friends easily.

_____ 10. I speak up for my own ideas, likes, and dislikes.

_____ 11. I am not hurt by others' opinions or attitudes.

_____ 12. I *do not* need praise to feel good about myself.

_____ 13. I feel good about others' good luck and winning.

_____ 14. I *do not* find fault with my family, friends, or others.

_____ 15. I *do not* feel I must always please others.

_____ 16. I am open and honest and not afraid of letting people see my real self.

_____ 17. I am friendly, thoughtful, and generous towards others.

_____ 18. I do not blame others for *my* problems and mistakes.

_____ 19. I enjoy being alone with myself.

_____ 20. I accept compliments and gifts without feeling uncomfortable or needing to give something in return.

_____ 21. I admit my mistakes and defeats without feeling ashamed or "less than."

_____ 22. I feel no need to defend what I think, say, or do.

_____ 23. I *do not* need others to agree with me or tell me I'm right.

_____ 24. I *do not* brag about myself, what I have done, or what my family has or does.

_____ 25. I *do not* feel "put down" when criticized by my friends or others.

_____ SELF-ESTEEM INDEX (sum of all scores)

TO FIND YOUR SELF-ESTEEM INDEX (SEI), simply add scores of all Self-Esteem Statements. The possible range of your Self-Esteem Index is from 0 to 100. Sound Self-Esteem is indicated by an SEI of 95 or more. Experience shows that any score under 90 is a disadvantage, a score of 75 or less is a serious disadvantage, and an SEI of 50 or less indicates a really hurting lack of Self-Esteem.

THE QUIET JOY OF THE RAINBOW

I suggest that each guest commemorate the day of arriving home from the Golden Door, because it is the start of a new life. In the early afternoon, take out your business calendar, study each page. I hope you too will want to commemorate the day you read the last page, close this book, and continue on your chosen path.

In the early afternoon, study each page as you might study your face. It's you—your time, your day. How you use all this determines your life. Look at the map of your life as it was. Now decide what to keep, what to discard, and what to change.

"Those who cannot remember the past are condemned to repeat it," said George Santayana. To plan your future, you must analyze your past. You must avoid the pitfalls of wishful thinking, the over-idealistic resolutions which we all hope for and rarely achieve, if you are to be realistic and successful. Consider the recent month you believe to be most typical. You are going to use this month to keep from floating off into rationalizations. Now underline each calendar entry as follows:

Black for anything you did that was a waste of yourself or your time, for anything that gave you neither pride nor satisfaction. Black for a period that just trickled away, was lost, and can't be ascribed to anything either active, creative, or contemplative.

Blue for duty, for earning and such necessities of life. Chores, responsibilities, and the like, those things which must be accomplished. The more you dislike them, the faster you should get them done.

Red for what you contributed to your health and physical well-being: a brisk walk, a set of tennis. Make daily deposits to your energy reserves for later withdrawal.

Green, for growth, your personal growth, every new dimension that has added—or will surely add—to the width and breadth of your life.

Plant any seed, it will sprout, germinate, grow. Remove the growth elements, it dies. So do we, each in our own way.

Lavender is for everything joyous. In my earliest childhood I almost wordlessly understood that healthy meant happy. So much laughter and song resounded around the evening bonfires of the New York Hiking Club, and, later, on the black sandy beaches of Tahiti. In my family's first months there in the South Seas, we rented a house with a tin roof. Close by was a waterfall. I remember the first time I awakened to the tropical rain pounding on our roof, and also to the gales of laughter emanating from the native women by the wet rocks beside the waterfall, where they pounded their washing with a stick. I can still recall my puzzlement: "How can they be laughing with the cold rain drumming down their fronts and backs?" It took me a while to realize that to primitive people laughter is a natural function like breathing. Afterward we lived in other small villages, and I always was amazed how easily laughter could be stirred among peoples who, by our standards, are so much less fortunate than we.

Today I seldom hear enough laughter, except among children at play, or from my rejuvenated guests, working out all those tensions on the exercise mats at the Golden Door.

SUNSHINE AND RAINBOW— PART OF YOUR DAILY COLOR BALANCE

Joy, like the bluebird of Maeterlinck, needs to be sought out. Joy can best be found at home but you have to create the right environment if joy is to thrive. For your health and growth and joy, every day should be rainbow-hued. Study your patterns. See where you can convert some of your blacks and some of your blues into reds, greens, and lavenders.

Be creative about it. Bicycling instead of driving will change some chores from black to red. Lunch in the park with a friend, instead of a hurried-up sandwich at your desk, turns out lavender. Of course, many blues are going to remain as they are. But you can intersperse them with reds and greens. They all serve to balance your day, providing more contrast and more pleasure to each alternating period.

Apply this principle to household duties, to office, and other tasks. Just as there needs to be an ecological balance in nature, so too there must be a balance in Man.

L'ENVOI

To restore my own balance, I never enter a new decade without a Wonder Weekend. As I have said, I was a June bride at fifty, a decision requiring several weekends. That was the same year my younger child became a freshman in high school. Every mother, even the busiest businesswoman, must spend time deliberating how she will function one day within an empty nest.

This year I took a number of weekends when my dear husband Vince decided that the differences which at first drew us together had become differences with which he no longer cared to cope. A few weeks before our sixth anniversary, he carefully explained how, all his life, he had looked forward to a quiet life. But, since obviously I had no intention of ever doing less, he wanted out.

I did love being married to him. I'm a tidy person who likes neat patterns. I had enjoyed my cozy, infinitely comfortable cocoon, and here I was being dropped back into the roaring mainstream. I loved being in love, to share, to mother and to care for someone who needs a different part of me and in return gives me a part of himself. My first inclination was to cry, to beg. But then I realized that I had no right to ask him to live my style of life. I was not willing to live his.

Each healing weekend did me good, sent me home more buoyant. Now, nine months after our parting, I can say that, had I known I was entering into a marriage of a six-year duration, I still would have agreed to it. It was a splendid six years for me and for Vince and both his and my children.

HOW TO READ YOURSELF
LIKE A BOOK

But back from me to you.

From year to year, save all your calendars, as I do. New Year's Day is a fine time to leaf through their pages. It will be like chapters from your autobiography, for there you are—yesterday, today, tomorrow. Note how transitory were the times of stress and sorrow. See how you remember so much more good than bad.

Review the habit patterns on which you have built your life to date. Save a few, and work to discard others so that you can fill your days with new being. You will sleepwalk through life if you repeat your days until there are none.

Use the present to prophesy your future.

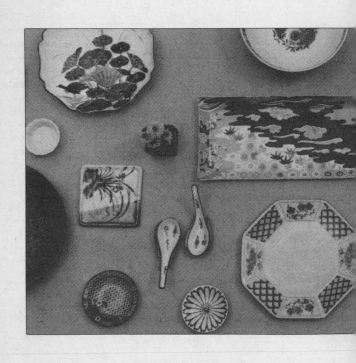

CHAPTER VIII

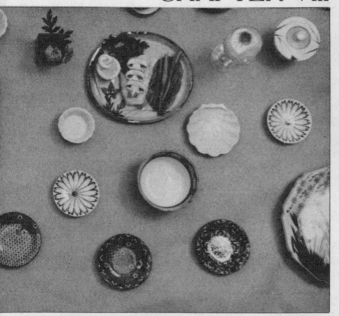

GLORIOUS EATING:
THE GOLDEN DOOR
WAY TO MAKE
FOOD YOUR FRIEND

Anyone who has ever lingered beside a newsstand knows how preoccupied Americans are with food and diet. One cannot help being aware of it—and confused about it as well. Do not deprecate the old adage "We are what we eat." It is all too true. The degree and quality of our health and, yes, the very quantity of our years depend upon our food. A motor without the proper fuel sputters and skips and finally stops. But our own organism lacks such fail-safe devices.

My goal will be to advise you how to pleasure yourself as you grow in your ability to balance your intake of proper food/fuel with your output of living energy. The secret, obviously, is to double your pleasure without doubling your calories, by emphasizing the psychological rather than the physical calorie. If you learn my lessons well, you'll have learned to discard your attitude of crime and punishment (i.e., the belief that it's a crime to eat, so you must punish yourself by dieting).

A GAME PLAN FOR LIFE

Appetite is nature's way of ensuring survival; loving food is part of loving life. Since eating is something you must do daily in order to sustain life, be demanding of the food you eat. It should taste very good and be very, very good for you. You must arrange a better way of eating that's both normal for you and consistent with your physical size and activity age.

My joy was immense when I read in early 1977 a report by the Senate Select Committee on Nutrition and Human Needs.* It confirmed what the Golden Door has been preaching during the past several decades.

TUNE UP
THE OLD-FASHIONED
HORN OF PLENTY

In effect, the report stated that Americans should go back to the old days and eat fruits, vegetables, and grains instead of relying on fats and sugars for 60 percent of their food energy. Our eating habits may be "as profoundly damaging to the nation's health as the widespread contagious diseases of the early part of the century." Rapidly increasing fat consumption has "been linked to six of the ten leading causes of death. . . . Too much fat, too much sugar or salt can be and are linked directly to heart disease, cancer, obesity and stroke, among other killer diseases."

In the 1977 edition consumers were asked to de-

*$2.30 is the cost of the second edition of the report, "Dietary Goals for the United States." Order from the Superintendent of Documents, U.S. Government Printing Office, Washington, DC 20402. Stock No. 052-070-04376-8.

crease their "refined and processed" sugar consumption to 15 percent instead of 24 percent of their total daily intake; total fats to 30 percent instead of 42 percent; salt to 3 grams instead of 6 grams; cholesterol to 300 milligrams from a previous average of 600. Since then, the revised edition has made certain changes: Americans now are being asked to reduce refined and processed sugars to 10 percent instead of 24 percent.

A new added goal is that one consume only as much energy as one expends.

The report still urges that increased consumption of fruits, vegetables, and grains substitute for fat and processed-sugar consumption. Americans are told they should eat less meat and more fish, and drink nonfat milk rather than whole milk.

The committee report is the first comprehensive statement by any branch of the federal government on the risks involved in the American diet, and most unexpected in a government document are the following two statements:

THE SENSUOUS
SHORT-ORDER COOK

From Mary Goodwin, public health nutritionist:

The pleasures of seeing, smelling, and tasting food that looks, smells, and tastes good, nourish the personality with sensuous experience even as the vitamins and minerals are making their contribution to the growth of bone and muscle. An awareness of real people preparing and serving the foods helps too.

Which is to say that if you eat enough precooked, frozen, reheated, foil-and-plastic packed lunches out of machines, part of you will starve to death.

YOUR X-RATED MENU

And from Dr. Bruno Bettelheim, noted child psychiatrist:

> Eating and being fed are intimately connected
> with our deepest feelings. They are the basic in-
> teractions between human beings on which rest
> all later evaluations of oneself, of the world, and of
> our relationship to it. Eating experiences condition
> our entire attitude to the world, not so much be-
> cause of how nutritious is the food we are given,
> but because of the feelings and attitudes with
> which it is given.

FOOD AS
LIFE ENHANCEMENT

Common sense is at last being applied. The concept
of living for life, rather than for death, is beginning to
make sense to the common man. Food values are expected to sustain life, rather than to diminish it.

Food in nature has its own ecological balance. The
closer to the natural state, the better for life. Each mile
traveled, each process, each nutrient removed or
added, how and for how long cooked, even the containers and what it's cooked in, all affect the life-
enhancing value of food/fuel.

FAD AND
FACT AND FANCIES

You've noticed that this chapter head uses the word
"food"—not "diet." And you've already gathered
why. I simply don't believe in denial, which diets entail.

Hear about crash diets from Cristina DeLorean, one of
the world's most beautiful and highly paid photo-
graphic models. "They make me sick," she says.

Her face was on the cover of eight national magazines
in one year and is seen repeatedly in current advertise-
ments for a leading cosmetics company. With all that

going for her, she was still battling our country's most pervasive beauty problem—overweight.

"I weighed too much for fashion modeling," she explains. "My face was okay, but I couldn't do clothes."

The nagging conviction that she was overweight frustrated her into a series of crash diets, all of them bad. "After a few days on one of those diets, I would begin to get dizzy and then start vomiting," she remembers. "I had to do something sensible."

One day she read an issue of *Town and Country* magazine devoted entirely to health and beauty spas. (Her picture was on the cover.) After studying the articles, she made a reservation at the Golden Door.

> I went expecting two weeks of aggravating diet and exercise. Within about four or five days I began to feel better than I had in a long, long time. By the second week, I felt better than I ever had in my whole life. I was a new person. It was a revelation that a well-balanced, low-calorie diet could taste good and be good for you.

When she left, Cristina took home Golden Door assets to share with her family. Her husband, John DeLorean, is an automobile designer and manufacturer. They have a four-year-old son, Zachary. Cristina notes:

> Modeling is hard work. It demands a lot of muscle control, and I have to be on my feet a good part of the day. I use Golden Door exercises to ease the pressure. No matter how tired I am when I come home from work, I get down on the floor and exercise. It gets my blood going and gives me my second wind. I feel great.

I'd no more urge a crash diet upon you than I would upon Cristina. What you must arrange is a better way of eating—one that's normal for you, as you are now, with your already established life-style.

DON'T GIVE YOUR BEST
SHOT TO A GAME
OF RUSSIAN ROULETTE

The so-called "newer" and "better" diets inevitably prove to be just a better way of deviling yourself with some new denial. Each new fad diet—like the others—is a game of Russian roulette. It may not kill you, but it produces new tensions and unhappiness by dictating that you sit in on a punishment game instead of a reward game.

I know whereof I speak because for many years I tried every new diet plan on my guests. Fortunately, one at last runs out of mistakes. What we have discovered with our guests at the Golden Door is an affirmative, creative way to *intensify* the pleasure you derive from sane quantities of really delectable food. The goal, after all, is not cessation of eating.

There is a folk tale—Romanian or Hungarian, depending upon who tells it—that says everything that needs to be said:

> A traveler was walking down a road when he saw a peasant leaning against a tree and weeping as if his heart had broken.
>
> "What is wrong?" the traveler asked. "Why are you weeping?"
>
> "My perfect horse!" the peasant sobbed. "It died!"
>
> "Ah. What made your perfect horse perfect?"
>
> For a while the peasant was too overcome to speak. Then at last he raised his head. "I worked with that horse for months. Oh, he cooperated so willingly! Every day he would eat a little less of my oats, less and less, until finally he got to the point where he became the perfect farm animal. He didn't have to eat at all. Nothing. Not a handful of oats, not a blade of grass.
>
> "And then—a catastrophe! An unimaginable misfortune! Just as he became perfect, he died."

CALCULATING THE
TOTAL CALORIE

The pleasure you experience from appropriate food can transform your looks, your health, and the overall stimulus that life brings you.

Food satisfies three basic needs:

1. Energy, to propel you
2. Delight, to motivate you
3. Nutrition, to build and maintain your body

Are your present eating habits truly fulfilling all these needs? Being active and exuberant, mixing out there in the world with all your ebullience and vitality is going to be vastly more worthwhile for you than anxiously counting calories. Never be intimidated by the word *calorie* and what it represents. It's only a specific measure of energy, after all, the amount of heat necessary to raise one gram of water one degree Centigrade. Caloric energy contained in a slice of bread is sufficient to bring nearly a quart of water to boil. And how's this for a makes-you-stop-and-think statistic: a pound of stored body fat has enough energy to boil more than thirteen gallons.

If you count only the physical calories in your diet you may always believe yourself hungry. But food also provides psychological calories. The magnificent San Diego Zoo utilizes diet pellets containing all the nutrients that each species of animal is known to need. Yet I was fascinated to see a special note at the bottom of the prescribed diet. It was labeled "For Delight," and listed apples, bananas, and certain fresh leaves. When I asked a zoo veterinarian what would happen if the animal didn't receive this special supplement, he said, "The coat becomes dull. Stools are irregular. Either there are almost no offspring or the offspring are deformed. The animal develops muscular problems. And, worst of all—he bites his keeper."

When you combine the physical calorie with the psychological calorie, you have what I call the Total Calorie, which I picture as a sort of iceberg. The visible top

10 percent is the physical calorie. It's supported by the invisible 90 percent, the psychological calorie.

If the calorie's impact were purely physical, Metrecal would be bigger than ITT. Need a refill? No problem. You'd mix some powder with water. When you ran out of energy, you'd buy some more at a Richfield or an Exxon, but you'd be a machine and not a human being. It is the psychological calorie that entices you, that is the mainstay of the advertising industry, be it television, radio, your daily newspaper, or your favorite magazine. When you get down to basics, your natural food is very basic. There are about fifty primary foods. Some dozen grains; another dozen legumes; certain families of fresh fruits and vegetables; dairy products and eggs; nuts; and your meats, poultry, and fish. From these come our machine-made food.

PRE-PACKAGED LOVE

As we know, food is love. Sold in the U.S. markets are about 60,000 different food items, some of them highly seductive creations, and almost all with varying sets of additives, chemicals, preservatives, etc. Each of these contribute to the diminishment of life rather than its enhancement. You make the decision as you reach out in the supermarket. With each box, or that jar, or can, ask yourself, "Is this my health, and my family's health, happiness, and long life?"

SUPER EATING FOR
LIFE ENHANCEMENT

Every calorie is filled with love, affection, memories. Do experience them all while you eat. Don't deprive yourself of any of your psychological calories. Never read or watch TV while eating, because the surrogate emotions evoked by reading or viewing will stand in the way of the satisfying emotional experience which should be part of your every meal. And if you are a workaholic like so many of us, it takes extra effort, but well worth it, to think food rather than work. So never ever eat at your desk. If you want to be truly satisfied, the lunch on a park bench or in a backyard garden is a lovely way to double your pleasure without doubling your calories. The peace that comes with a good meal is not derived from the meal alone. The break in tension is from the change in tension rather than the fact that you've given your stomach something to do.

Since eating is an act of intake, you are open and vulnerable not only to food but to suggestion. Hence the business or social lunch where, with your defenses down, you can easily be talked into something you would rather not do. Since Biblical times food has been rightly associated with sharing, with opening up. If you know that the pleasure of sharing with partner, family, or friends awaits you during the evening, it is ever so much easier to limit yourself to a small breakfast and a very modest lunch.

Food takes care of emotional needs that are real and profound. By all means make food your friend—but by no means your *only* friend. Really serious weight problems usually belong to the men and women who forsake all other gratifications for those of the table.

YOUR CUSTOM-MADE
CALORIE TOTAL

People often approach me to ask, "What is the right diet for me?" as if I carried diet regimens like color swatches to be quickly matched to the proper person.

The only satisfactory answer to this question is a complex answer. In her book, *Between Heaven and Earth,* my friend Laura Huxley suggests that you cannot determine the right diet for yourself until you first have answered questions such as these:

Where do you live? How old are you? What kind of job do you have?

Is your sex life satisfactory? How do you feel toward

yourself? With whom do you eat? What is your last thought at night? Are you in love? What is your first thought in the morning?

Do you have children? Is the intensity of your emotional feeling markedly different before and after a meal? Is your sense of smell a keen guide, or do you hardly notice it? Do you breathe consciously sometimes?

Do you meditate? Do you have a totally satisfactory relationship with one or more persons? Are you now living in a condition physically, psychologically, or emotionally stressful?

Laura concludes: "Your answers to these and other questions, coordinated with your genetic heritage and chemical analysis, are basic to your choice of diet and of food supplements."*

LESS IS MORE

Over the years at the Golden Door we have perfected a variety of techniques for making a relatively small amount of food immensely satisfying. You can enhance your enjoyment by following them.

1. *Less is more* if you continue to eat whatever you genuinely like. If you really detest something—even though somebody has told you it's a wonder food—don't eat it. Especially in times of stress, it's important that you retain familiar flavors, textures, and cooking fragrances at mealtime.

Hold onto all your pet recipes, but serve the "main course" on the salad plate and the salad on the dinner plate. If steak is a dinner favorite, the accompaniment should be something lean like zucchini. Reserve baked potatoes for fish or soufflé nights. If spaghetti is the side dish, it's time for clear soup, green salad, and a dessert of fruit. When there's a birthday cake, all the other courses should be low in calories. This way you can eat

*Between Heaven and Earth. Laura Archera Huxley. New York: Farrar, Straus, and Giroux, 1975.

what you've always been fond of and yet not add un-
wanted pounds. It's all merely a matter of balancing
total intake.

2. *Less is more* when you consciously eat in very
agreeable surroundings and without distractions. Infre-
quently, I hear a Golden Door guest complain of hunger.
I first check to see if she has eaten in her room. Almost
invariably, she has. Gulping down almost-unnoticed
food while reading or sitting in bed is no way to savor
it.

At home, standing by the refrigerator and eating is
one of the best means of getting fat without enjoying
food. And newspapers and television are dreadful
mealtime partners, literally specters at the feast. All
these distractions mean that you'll entertain only a mo-
mentary sort of gullet pleasure which doesn't last long;
soon you're hungry again.

When you're eating alone, favor yourself with the
sensuous delights of flowers, a cheerful tray, and your
best china. Carry your food out of the kitchen and into
a harmonious setting.

3. *Less is more* when you eat with agreeable people,
whether family or friends. Conversation and companionship make food seem even more satisfying. Always
take care at table to keep all conversation upbeat and
interesting. Dinnertime, usually, is the only hour of the
day when the entire family can sit down to share a
happy experience. Make it happy for everyone, including yourself.

4. *Less is more* when you open your senses in new
directions. Normal as it is to find gratification in food, it
is dangerous to depend on it for most of your rewards.

Find instead rewarding involvements. These can be
even more satisfying than food, for the soul needs feeding even more than the body.

Begin by scheduling simple daily pleasures for yourself—a new hairdo, a scarf, a record, a get-away-from-
it-all swim—things you can arrange casually. Instead of
dreaming of exquisite menus and Brillat-Savarin fetes,
settle for a new class, a new book, a concert, or a

movie. Assume a gourmet attitude toward *all* of living, and you'll have little trouble adhering to your new diet plan.

And consider this: When you're uncomfortable or bored, your body relays signals of dissatisfaction which are often mistaken for hunger. Actually, you then may need a change of pace—a splash of cold water on your face, a quick brisk walk, or just a tiny, healthful snack to lift your blood sugar and renew your energy.

As for true hunger, it can come to be your friend if you learn to associate the sensation with good looks and vitality and with pride in your body. See in each dish the quality of your life.

BEGINNING YOUR FOOD PLAN

Before you can improve your eating patterns you must be thoroughly aware of them.

1. TAKE A CLOSE LOOK AT HOW YOU EAT. For three days write down everything, how much, when, where, with whom. Do you nibble and snack, or eat one big meal; if you snack, is it from the time you begin to prepare dinner until bedtime? Do you dine out often? Do you eat with the family, or from a solitary tray? In the kitchen, bedroom, dining room, living room? While you read or watch TV? In the beginning count every physical calorie so you'll have an accurate picture of your intake—per meal and per day. (At any bookstore and many newsstands you can buy one of those inexpensive paperbacks listing the calories contained in standard servings of almost every imaginable food. My favorite is *Calories and Carbohydrates* by Barbara Kraus.)

2. SELECT YOUR ACTIVITY AGE. Look closely at both sides of the energy equation: Calorie *intake* (ideally) equals energy *output*. Laborers, for example, and many teen-agers and professional athletes who burn up terrific amounts of energy in their daily activities can consume five or six thousand calories a day—two or

three times as much as the average thirty-five-year-old American would dare—without gaining weight.

If you eat as much as you always have and don't step up your exercise, you'll add fat. If you heedlessly allow yourself to grow older with your intake at the same level, the gradual changes in your output eventually will unbalance your system. So think. Even if you're young now, by allowing yourself to gain a pound a year at each Christmas dinner you'll be twenty pounds over-weight when you blow out the forty or so candles on your cake.

To be more specific: if you consume an excess of only ninety-six calories a day (the equivalent of one slice of bread), in five years you could conceivably be fifty pounds overweight. In contrast, the weight gain could have been prevented if only twenty-five minutes of brisk walking had been added to each day. And don't forget that the benefits of exercise continue long after you have stopped moving. So do walk a few extra blocks and up the stairs before sitting in that office chair, both in the morning and again at lunch. Walking a brisk mile each day for thirty-five days is a simple way to lose a pound—walk more and you will lose more. Those who are overweight have an even greater potential for losing weight since it takes more energy to move two hundred pounds than one hundred pounds.

Your body is not a statistic. That's why I'm not includ-ing a "Recommended Calories Per Day by Weight and Age" chart, nor a "Recommended Weight by Height and Age." I don't believe in them. The mirror is your surest measuring stick, and the bathroom scale is your best daily gauge.

HIDDEN CALORIES STRIPPED BARE

One vividly graphic way to understand calories so well that you may never again have to try to count any has been developed at the Golden Door. Once a week we display a table of *Foods in 100-calorie Portions.* The contrast between the quantities provides a dramatic demonstration. One tablespoon of mayonnaise is the caloric equivalent of two cups of tomato juice, something to ponder when you mix your own salad dressing. And dessert lovers can think this over: a whole papaya, or two and one-half cups of watermelon, equal two tablespoons of heavy cream.

Look at the chart, and then look in your own refrigerator. What startling inequities do you see? Setting up a 100-calorie display on your own dining-room table is a painless and emphatic way to teach children about good vs. junk food, or to spur on some family member who should lose weight. The Golden Door's display, and this book's 100-calorie chart, are the work of our Shirley Matson, as is the additives chart (pages 278–79).

FOODS IN 100-CALORIE PORTIONS

Food	Approximate Measure	Approximate Weight
Almonds	2 tbsp.	1½ ounces
Asparagus	3½ cups	
Banana	1 medium	6 ounces
Beef, lean, ground		1¾ ounces
Bean sprouts	3 cups	
Beans, green, fresh	3 cups	¾ pound
Bran	¾ cup	
Bran muffin	1 small	
Broccoli, fresh	2½ cups	1¼ pounds
Bread, whole wheat	2 slices	
Butter	1 tbsp.	
Cantaloupe	1 small	1½ pounds
Carrots		¾ pound
Celery		1¾ pounds
Cereal (oatmeal, cooked)	⅔ cup	
Cereal (Grape Nuts)	¼ cup	
Cheese, Cheddar		1 ounce
Cheese, Parmesan, grated	3½ tbsp.	
Cheese, Swiss		1 ounce

Chicken, white meat	½ cup	2 ounces
Crackers (Rye Krisp)	4 crackers	
Cucumbers	5 cups	2½ pounds
Cream, heavy	2 tbsp.	
Egg, whole, large	1¼ eggs	
Fish, fillet of sole		4½ ounces
Fish, tuna, packed in water		3 ounces
Honey	5 tbsp.	
Lettuce, romaine	20 8″ leaves	
Margarine	1 tbsp.	
Mayonnaise	1 tbsp.	
Mushrooms	5 cups	¾ pound
Nuts, Brazil	4 nuts	
Nuts, macadamia	6 nuts	½ ounce
Nuts, walnut	2 tbsp.	
Orange juice, fresh	1 cup	8 ounces
Orange segments	1 cup	
Papaya	1 whole	¾ pound
Peanuts	2 tbsp.	0.6 ounce
Peanut butter	1 tbsp.	0.6 ounce
Potato, baked	1 small	5 ounces
Popcorn, plain	2½ cups	
Prunes	6 medium	
Raisins	¼ cup	1 ounce
Raspberries	1¼ cups	
Rice, brown, cooked	½ cup	
Spinach, fresh, untrimmed	4½ cups	1¼ pounds
Strawberries, fresh	2 cups	
Sunflower seeds	2 tbsp.	¾ ounce
Tomatoes	3 medium	1 pound
Tomato juice	2 cups	
Watermelon, diced, fresh	2½ cups	
Wheat germ	¼ cup	
Zucchini	5 cups	1¼ pounds

3. RELATE YOUR INTAKE TO YOUR BODY SIZE. The logic of this is impressed upon us very early when someone first reads us the story of "Goldilocks and the Three Bears". . .

In a neat little cottage in the midst of a deep woods there once lived three bears. One was a great big daddy bear, one was a middle-sized mama bear, and one was a wee little baby bear.

One morning Mother Bear made a big batch of porridge for breakfast. She filled a great big bowl for daddy bear, a middle-sized bowl for her middle-sized self, and a wee little bowl for baby bear. . . .

I'm appalled at the civilized nonsense called "portion control," a measured serving for the mythical average man. This evil is practiced in every school, restaurant, and hospital in the country, and in most homes. A flagrant illustration of this was told me by Stephen McClintock, the physiologist who administered my stress test to me:

"I'm six feet, six inches tall, and in the Army where you line up to be served, I followed a four-foot-six soldier. No matter how I pleaded for food, I was told, 'Everyone is treated equally in the Army.' So I got skinnier and skinnier and my messmate got fatter and fatter."

SNACKS ARE THE ENEMY

Vivid Bess Myerson, thirty years ago the nation's stunning beauty queen, and now our leading advocate for consumer protection, has developed a personal approach. "Snacks are the enemy," she says, knowing exactly where she stands in this controversy.

Bess is a busy woman, and her remarkable career continues to embrace the widest range of roles: TV and radio commentator; newspaper and magazine writer/editor; lecturer, teacher, and consultant to consumer and industry associations. As Commissioner of Consumer Affairs for New York City, she pioneered many consumer-protection programs which have been adopted by numerous cities.

She makes the point that people as busy and on-the-go as most of us today have two basic problems—to find the time to eat, and to find the willpower to eat correctly. "It isn't easy in our snack society," she says:

"Grabbing a bite to eat" may do wonders for our daily timetables but it certainly doesn't do much for our health—or our hips. That kind of tension—which is a sign of our times—can unbalance a diet. The Golden Door helped me get the balance back. Its good food and good sense about food can strengthen even the most lagging of willpowers. It isn't enough for any of us to know about food and nutrition and additives, and the value of exercise, and the rules of health that we break at our own peril. We also have to know the places and opportunities which make it easier for us to do more than just think about those things, while we are running around and snacking ourselves into trouble.

I looked for those places and opportunities—and I found one. Behind the Golden Door, you might say. My willpower is doing nicely, thank you.

4. MAKE YOUR OWN FOOD PLAN. Tailor a program to suit yourself; go on making alterations and adjustments till it fits you exactly.

My lawyer friend John Rhoades developed his own individualistic slant on dieting:

"From Monday to Friday I eat sparingly: a light breakfast, not too much lunch, and very little dinner. I promise myself that from Friday night until Sunday night I can eat anything I want. All week I look forward to the bonus weekend when I can drink my beer and eat Mexican food and lasagna and all that." Certainly not a utopian diet plan but, if it works for him, that's all that counts. Let me add that John, who lives by the sea, runs three miles every morning on the beach and takes a quick swim before work. He weighs less today than when he joined the Navy years ago.

5. DON'T BE IMPATIENT. Don't be too ambitious. Your eating habits took years to form. Long-established habits can't be altered overnight, nor should they be.

6. SELECT A MANAGEABLE GOAL. You remember my tricks of a ten-percenter: eat 10 percent less, exercise 10 percent more, and think 10 percent more. It's a very low-pressure game that nevertheless will bring you out on top at year's end, like a sound conservative investment. The thinking calls for you to outwit yourself in little ways. Examples: make 4 ounces of morning orange juice into 8 ounces by diluting with 50 percent water. Begin a later-day meal with a bulky low-calorie salad or a clear soup.

The result, as I have figured out, is that if you eat 10 percent fewer calories all year, you can have a few weekend bacchanalias and still weigh less than you would otherwise.

7. REMEMBER THE PSYCHOLOGICAL CALORIE, particularly at the end of the day. When we discuss their "take-out" plan before guests leave the Golden Door, I always question them closely about their pre-dinner habits and usually make major changes there.

If you come home starved and you still have dinner to prepare, recognize that your entire food plan is in peril, for the degree of tension of the day will carry on through dinner and the evening unless you take a deliberate action to down-gear to a new, more appropriate evening speed. Now indeed you need "the pause that refreshes," not a Coke or a drink but a minute or two of jumping rope in your office, and then a tiny snack in your car as you drive home. Or in your living room, looking out, think cozy thoughts while you munch an apple and nibble on a few nuts and dried fruits. As you contemplate the third/third of your day, picture the surge in your body's blood sugar when your energy begins its circle of renewal.

If your body has been inactive while your mind has been whirling, you must expect that it will take effort to reunite body and mind and to return them to functioning at the same harmonious speed. I have a plan that works well for me, and my guests tell me it has proven equally successful for them.

I begin the act of unwinding by stopping at the market. Since I plan dinner at the breakfast table, it takes only five minutes to pick up what I will need for that night, for I buy just the right amount for the precise size, activity age, and number of people I will feed, plus whatever I lack to prepare breakfast and/or lunch the following day.

Since I concentrate on life-enhancing rather than on life-diminishing foods, the whole process is simple: first to the produce department for the best and freshest; then to the milk, eggs, and cheese section; a brief stop to pick up some grains and dried legumes; and perhaps a moment to select the freshest of the fish and poultry.

Once at home I empty my grocery bags on the kitchen counter. Since I never have to put anything away, I have time for the all-important transition period of exercise, shower (very hot and then very cold), and change of clothes that spells relaxation. Never go directly from daytime work to the kitchen, to work on the evening meal. If you do, you will find little pleasure in either the food preparation or in dinner; they will be mere preliminaries to getting the dishes done. When I return to the kitchen, content and relaxed, there is no need to ponder which vegetables and fruits should be used first, since we'll be eating the food at once. My kitchen has no need for a gigantic refrigerator, and when I open the fridge door I don't have to puzzle over what to do with the leftovers—there are none. I know from personal experience that my empty refrigerator is one of my very best friends.

THE CALORIE GAME: FIGURING THE PERCENTAGES

Once you have probed your eating habits (and certain other personal tendencies), we'll assume you've decided to reduce your intake of physical calories.

A good rule of thumb when combining food and exercise facts is to remember the estimate that a pound of fat is worth 3,500 calories. In figuring out your own weight-loss schedule, you may assume that for every 3,500 calories you either don't swallow, or burn away, you can eliminate one pound of real fat—not just a pound of water that will return the next day.

By trimming off just 100 of your daily calories, you can lose that full pound of fat in 35 days. Slow, but you do need nutrients and the satisfactions of the Total Calorie. If you cut back too far, you may feel malnourished, uneasy, and unhappy. That's why at the Golden Door, where the most controlled circumstances prevail, the weight-loss diet is rarely permitted to drop below a daily average of 800 calories, 1,000 if you are over 5'4", and 600 if you are under 5'. (See menus, pages 306–385) If you're at home and taxed by the usual mundane stresses and you're a middle-sized, middle-aged female, you shouldn't let your daily total slip below 1,250 calories. For a middle-sized, middle-aged male, 2,000 calories often is the desirable minimum. Let exercise do its share in the weight-loss program. It is a fact that it is easier for a man to lose weight on more food than it is for a woman. Because of his size, a man requires more calories just to maintain minimal body functions. Women have a higher proportion of fat cells, and consequently a lower proportion of cell-mass (muscle mass) than men; and as we age, watch out!—for the total cell-mass continues to decrease as the years increase.

TIMELY, TIDY, TINY—
THE NEWEST WEIGHT CHART

Today I was gratified by a very small thing—one of those tiny booklets you buy at supermarket checkstands (*Count Your Calories,* a Dell Purse Book), its back dedicated to a sensible age/weight/calorie chart for men and women 18 to 75. How different from the old "average recommended height and weight charts" that used to be featured in so many of the magazines. When information of this sort from the Food and Nutrition Board of the National Academy of Sciences is distributed by a mass-medium publication costing 49 cents, it's a welcome step forward. It reflects more widespread awareness that our calorie-energy requirements are constantly declining.

The energy requirements of the body depend on the basal metabolic rate which is affected by both the degree of physical activity and the body size. The basal metabolic rate is the measurement of energy output when one is in a state of complete rest, and it depends on the total cell-mass. To simplify it all, think of the cell-mass as that which consumes energy, speeding you up, and fat cells as those which store energy, slowing you down.

HOW TO
SQUEEZE A CALORIE

A proper balance of vigorous exercise and both the correct amounts and quality of food is a must. Whatever your age, you need to begin now.

At the Golden Door we apportion our calories differently from just about every other authority on food. That's because we want you to save your precious calories and to schedule Lucullan rewards for the hour of the day when you need them most. We want you to ensure yourself the most gratification, the most relaxation, the most opportunity for communicating meaningfully with someone else as you dine. In other words, we advise you to hold out for hedonism of a mild sort.

The Golden Door achieves splendid results from its 1,250-calories-a-day regimen, yet this allotment is far more generous than that advocated in *The Woman Doctor's Diet for Women*. Author Dr. Barbara Edelstein, 5'4", who once weighed in at 180, recommends a daily caloric intake below 1,000 calories—sometimes even less than 600. "Anything above 1,200," she says flatly, "is a thing of the past."

HOW TO HANG ONE ON,
CALORICALLY SPEAKING

As prelude to explanation of the Golden Door's daily apportionment of approximately 1,250 calories, I'm going to surprise you with my advice about the matter of emotional eating:

Go on, eat emotionally! I urge it if you have just undergone an experience that leaves you feeling unsure of yourself or very tense. It's natural to want to adjust your menu priorities and throw the lion's share of your day's calories to whatever meal comes along next. That meal will make you feel loved. Make sure you're eating something fairly light, nothing that will churn in your perhaps agitated stomach or feel like deadweight there. Now is the time for that long-avoided ice-cream sundae or that airy, melt-in-your-mouth French pastry. Or a little chicken Kiev.

Knowing you are about to splurge at once, and being secure in the knowledge that something so supportive is coming your way soon, you of course will precede your self-indulgent meal with a ten-minute exercise tension break; emotionally, you can afford to do so. And in this manner you will be bolstered by one good friend, bodily movement, even before you look for solace from another good friend, food.

BREAKFAST IS PRELIMINARY
TO THE MAIN EVENT

Allotting 10 or 20 percent for breakfast may not seem like much, but these days who has time for more? If you're allowing yourself 1,250 calories for the full day, this will amount to some 125 or 250 for the morning meal—just enough to lift the blood sugar and start you off. (If you're exercising on the morning pattern, as explained in the Movement chapter (page 19), thirty minutes of satisfying exercise movement will get you started. You've already feasted on oxygen!)

A number of people declare that a large breakfast gives them an early-day high that hangs on and on and on, as if they had been charged with 250 volts. Certainly there's no reason for you to be married forever to a skimpy one. But the Golden Door's very successful weight-loss plan always has been predicated on just a few morning calories. You've rested all night, you have unwound, and you don't need a lot of stoking in the morning. The whole day is ahead—a marvelous blank page on which you can fill in anything you want.

Yes, I've read the late, influential Adelle Davis's recommendation of big breakfasts. She argued so persuasively that for a week I drew up elaborate breakfast menus—but to no one's benefit, for in my house, and quite possibly in yours, there's no one around on weekday mornings to relish a sizable meal. How many people are disposed to linger and chat in the mornings?

The classic Golden Door breakfast is very simple: a heaping tablespoon of miller's bran (the kind you buy in the health-food store or feed store); two heaping tablespoons of wheat-germ flakes; and a heaping tablespoon of raisins. Sprinkle with cinnamon,* add one-half cup of low-fat milk. That's it. Just as we need to brush our teeth to eliminate plaque, and brush our heart with great gobs of oxygen, so must we brush our insides. This we do with a stiff fibre brush. It is important that it have the desired effect daily. When it doesn't, increase the amount of bran to two tablespoons; chop dried prunes soaked overnight or figs into the mixture; you might even replace the low-fat milk with prune juice.

OUT OF ORDURE

When I heard that Dr. Denis Burkitt, the bran man, was to speak at U.S. Naval Hospital in San Diego, I hurried over.

Dr. Burkitt's topic was Human Ordure—once a respectable diagnostic specialization among doctors.

*Buy it, or any other spice, from a fancy kitchen shop, and you will multiply the usual flavor. Extract every iota of taste from every meal.

Burkitt is making it respectable again by presenting it in his wonderfully witty way.

From this British physician's viewpoint, two of the worst calamities in history were universal education and the invention of the milling machine. Tensions set off by restrictive sitting caused schoolchildren to pass hard, bullet-like stools (healthy stools are soft and float). Milling removed from cereal grain the fibre that would have prevented the problem. Solution: Bran for breakfast. A must.

Burkitt blames low-fibre diets for most colon difficulties, which often lead eventually to cancer of the colon. He says the same culprit is responsible for hemorrhoids, varicose veins, diverticulitis, and even diabetes.

The Burkitt theory that particularly fascinated me related specifically to cancer of the colon. The good doctor points out that this grave problem of civilized man is almost unknown in primitive societies. His theory is that the natural carcinogens in our foods (and the myriad combinations made possible by technology as applied to food manufacturing) when deposited in pockets in our colons and incubated at a body temperature of 98.8 for a week may well be the culprit.

Obviously, I agree with the current emphasis on his fibrous foods. Perhaps I'm more easily convinced because even in 1940 we ground our grains immediately before baking and then served and sold our home-baked bread to our guests.

If you have some idiosyncratic inability to tolerate bran, use whole-grain breads. If you are happier with more breakfast, then half a cantaloupe and ½ ounce of Monterey Jack cheese on half a slice of homemade wheat toast; or a grated apple with cinnamon, raisins, and a few chopped nuts; or ½ cup yogurt with wheat germ and a few raisins; or a cracker spread with cottage cheese and cinnamon slipped under the broiler; all can be a prelude to some invention of your own.

WAKE IT AND SHAKE IT

At the Golden Door, I tell my guests they must expect to be tired on awaking. After all, they have lain quietly for eight hours, now obviously it is time to move. The stimulant needed is exercise rather than any form of coffee or tea.

In any event, your breakfast should include some form of substantial whole grain, for the B-complex vitamins and the indispensable trace minerals. The whole grains should be as close to their natural state as possible (remember, bread once was called the Staff of Life).

The Golden Door food plan leans heavily on raw fresh fruits and vegetables and natural whole grains. All of these contain as many extraordinary unknown life-giving substances as they do known ones.

At Rancho La Puerta as well as the Golden Door, it cannot be said that the serving of fibrous foods is enjoying a revival. At neither place did they ever go into a decline.

COFFEE, TEA, AND THEE

Sip your tea without sugar. If coffee is your drink, you'll want to be sure to replace it with a coffee substitute or a decaffeinated version because you'll not be needing stimulants. Even decaffeinated isn't entirely without caffeine. A California State University, Los Angeles, study found 3 milligrams in 5 ounces, compared to 58–70 milligrams in instant coffee. More than brand names, brewing accounted for fluctuations in the coffees tested. Instant coffee contained about two-thirds as much caffeine as perked, and percolator coffee about two-thirds as much as the high-scoring dripolator variety. One-minute tea at best has about 19 milligrams in 4.55 ounces; the amount can be nearly doubled if tea is brewed from 3 to 5 minutes. Japanese green tea bags tested lower than any U.S. tea, and a bit lower than some chocolate drinks.

Among adults, coffee may or may not be a black-dyed villain, although there is shattering new evidence linking it to birth defects. Certainly it has been held responsible for digestive upsets and rapid heartbeat as well as insomnia in many persons.

LUNCHEON, YOUR SLICK
NOONTIME CAPER

YOUR APPETITE SPOILER (planned snacks). Remember your mother telling you, "Don't eat anything before dinner; it will spoil your appetite!"? Well, Mom was right. And we recommend systematic appetite spoilers before each noon and evening meal. The appetite spoiler will begin to raise the blood-sugar level, sending impulses to inform the brain that the body has been fed. This process requires a full thirty to forty minutes. After a low-calorie meal it's desirable to recognize the process which takes place. Then you can silently be aware of your rising blood-sugar level and know that in just so many minutes you won't feel hungry. The spoiler can contribute a head start and shorten the gnawing gap between mealtime and its resultant satisfaction.

A FEW EXERCISE LICKS THAT SHOW PROMISE. Lifting your blood-sugar level cuts your appetite but doesn't break your tension. To be properly receptive for luncheon or any meal, you must be relaxed. At noontime, this is where your brief ten-minute (longer if possible) exercise stint comes in. Besides relaxing you, the brief exercise I recommend at this time (is there no end to my double-dyed plotting for your own good!) releases glucagon into your bloodstream; this energy hormone reduces appetite.

YOUR LUNCHEON STRETCHERS. Here again, 250 or 375 calories for lunch isn't generous, but you can make it seem so.

It's imperative to take luncheon in two courses. At home, lead off with an appetizer—your appetite spoiler. It can be a serving of berries, or celery stuffed with pot cheese, or a bowl of consommé, or a tomato-and-onion salad served with almost no dressing—just something low-calorie to set off the physiological process. Wait fifteen minutes. Make some phone calls. Open your junk mail. Inspect your garden.

If you work in an office, have your spoiler just as you leave to take your lunch hour. Nibble sunflower seeds and a small apple, or eat a half-cup of plain yogurt. Then walk to the restaurant. If you have spent 75 calories on the appetite spoiler, you still have 175 to 300 calories for the rest of your luncheon.

And now the luncheon, itself.

Each noon, crisp up your energy with a different and large mixed vegetable salad. Top it with one of our dressings, or one of your own. That might be oil and wine vinegar, or lemon juice, with seasonings and a grated, hard-cooked egg; yogurt with curry powder, salt, and pepper; yogurt with crumbled blue cheese, plus seasonings. When vegetables are truly fresh, little more is necessary. I love to add a bit of French mustard or horseradish; great salad herbs are fresh or dried mint, tarragon, oregano, rosemary, or basil.

Besides the salad you'll want a low-calorie protein: an omelette or assorted low-fat cheeses; broiled chicken without the skin; fish, or veal. But no luncheon meats, with their nitrates and other preservatives.

UPFRONT WITH YOUR TASTE BUDS. My own quick low-calorie luncheon is cottage cheese with a zinger of fresh Mexican salsa with lots of fresh tomatoes and cilantro chopped in. This satisfies me because I happen to adore Mexican food. It might not appeal to you. But it illustrates a point which has been made about the satisfaction derived from strong flavors. If I ate bland cottage cheese alone, my appestat still might have a dangerous reading. For some people, it is wise to begin any meal with a few mouthfuls of the most flavorful food on the table, even with a bit of a sweet.

OUTWIT YOUR WAITER. Eating in restaurants calls for other strategies. Read only the top of the menu, where the intriguing appetizers are listed. Order one with negligible calories, such as a slice of melon or a shrimp cocktail. When it arrives, tell the waiter it looks so good that you'd like him to bring you yet a second appetizer. The second dish can be much higher in calories. Such departures from routine usually disconcert a busy establishment—so you'll surely be able to settle in for a fifteen- or twenty-minute wait for your second course to arrive and your body to react to the fact that you have eaten.

It's fun. You'll sample all sorts of piquant things you haven't eaten in years. But don't undo your good work by stumbling over the rolls and butter on your table. If you can afford the calories in something like a thin slice of pumpernickel toast, put that slice on your butter plate and ask the waiter to remove the tempting remainder.

OLIVER TWIST REVISITED— DARING TO ASK FOR LESS

You may notice one point missing from my restaurant strategy: I used to advocate leaving 10 percent of your food on the plate. This advice I still see reprinted elsewhere from time to time, but in light of the national power shortage and the world food shortage I can no longer bring myself to say it. Instead, I think restaurants should be discouraged from being so prodigal. A Chicago-area nutritionist who believes as I do has a special "package" for travelers who must dine out a lot. She includes a bit of assertiveness training so people will not be intimidated by waiters and will boldly speak out for smaller portions; dressings and sauces on the side; skim instead of whole milk; and no cold cuts or preformed turkey tossed into chef's salads.

Lunch over and you still think you're hungry? Look at your watch, know it takes some forty-five minutes for your body to register that you have eaten to satisfaction.

DINNER, NOURISHMENT WITH A FLOURISH

This is the time for claiming your just rewards. It is the gold star for doing all that was expected of you throughout the day. It's certainly not the time to contend with a punishing diet. If the woman who prepares the meal can't eat it, the child within her is going to feel deprived. With no food to enjoy while her dinner partners are savoring theirs with gusto, she may pick at people. That's why I implore you to save 70 percent of your daily calories—875 of your 1,250—for a dinner you can approach with good-humored expectation.

NO WHINING WHILE DINING

On one of my lecture tours I remember spending a lovely day with a very congenial woman. I thought, "Isn't she nice. I just wish she lived in San Diego so we could be friends." And then I had dinner at her home.

Perhaps because I was there, and had just delivered a talk about the importance of weight reduction, she had served herself hummingbird-sized portions of everything. And, perhaps because she felt denied, all she did throughout the entire meal was to pick at her children. At the end of twelve minutes, when the children stood up and said, "So long, Mom. So long, Pop. Gotta run," I felt like going too.

MAKING YOUR
CALORIES S·T·R·E·T·C·H

Dinner should be a cleverly staged ritual. By serving as many courses as you can contrive, one at a time, on as many appealing small dishes as you can assemble, you stretch out the presentation of food, dramatize the pleasure everyone extracts from it, and create an illusion of opulence. At the Golden Door I insist the waitresses give service that anywhere else would be considered terrible—attentive but poky. Each course comes at widespread intervals, and dessert never is served until at least forty-five minutes after we first sit down. All this ceremony makes a meal more satisfying. It improves conversation, too. I have never had a guest get up after dinner and say she was still hungry; the secret is in the forty-five minutes. Try it tonight!

Before the evening meal, serve an extravaganza of hors d'oeuvres, 50-calorie raw vegetable snacks with a low-calorie dip. To accompany the *crudités,* add a champagne glass of something low-calorie and chilled, such as fruit juice over crushed ice, a wine spritzer, or a bit of champagne with orange juice.

Lastly—and with a flourish—serve dessert. Ripe fresh fruit, beautifully presented, or a frosty, fresh-fruit sherbet will satisfy your craving for sweets.

If you're single or if you are alone for an evening, switch luncheon and dinner by taking your main meal at noon. Celebrate it with a friend. Let dinner that evening be the simple salad and protein meal others had at lunch—who wants to eat a seven-course dinner alone?

SEVEN WAYS TO CURTAIL CALORIES

Here are **7** Golden Door techniques to help you cut weight sensibly and permanently:

1. SCHEDULE YOUR DELIGHTS. How you distribute your daily intake can be crucial to the success or failure of your food plan. Save your calories for the time of day you most need them—when they can give you the most pleasure, the most relaxation, and the most opportunity to communicate with someone else.

2. LET'S DECONTROL "PORTION CONTROL." Decorate your table with flowers and candles, not with food. Remember, no family-style "everything in the center of the table" platters. Serve only from the kitchen. If you do it properly, a five-year-old could tell which portion is intended for which person: the big portion to the person who wants to be bigger, and the small for whoever yearns to be smaller. Remember, garnishes both please and fool the eye, making portions seem larger. Pile on the parsley and mushrooms and lemon wedges.

3. DISH UP YOUR MEALS WITH A DIFFERENCE. If you inherited your great-aunt's Wedgwood or your grandmother's Spode, it's possible you still can replace a teacup in your pattern and no one will be the wiser.

This is very soothing to china collectors and other tradi-
tionalists, but upsetting to anyone who considers that
the manufacturers of dishware have arbitrarily been
turning out the same-size dinner plates for over a century.

Scramble the sequence you usually use for serving.
Again, remember to reverse the sequence: serve the
salad (the lowest calorie food) on the dinner plate and
the entrée (the highest calorie food) on the bread-and-
butter dish. Serve dessert in demitasse cups, to be
eaten with demitasse spoons. Or you can do as I did the
year I turned fifty: replace all your dinner china with the
smallest possible luncheon set.

4. EAT INEFFICIENTLY—PLAY WITH YOUR FOOD.
Stretch out mealtimes for as long as possible, especially
at dinner. Discard that well-remembered admonition
from our childhood: "Don't play with your food."

Play with your food!

Why? Try inviting a thin friend for lunch. She'll pick at
her plate, cut all her food into weird shapes, move it
from the left side of the dish to the right, and only after
a lot of handling will she put anything into her mouth.
Then she will chew and chew. After your dish has been
empty for five minutes, she might exclaim, "Oh! I'm
keeping you waiting," and leave some of her food on
the plate.

Then invite your fattest friend to luncheon and watch.
You'll behold a model of efficiency. Cut, stab, lift, chew,
all in a single motion. There goes one mouthful of food
after another. She doesn't know it, but she might take
in four times as much as the thin person does while
performing the same amount of touching and chewing,
and getting not one whit more satisfaction.

You know how this behavior originated. Mothers always applaud the quick, tidy eater faultlessly perched in
the little high chair, each mouthful disappearing with no
to-do. And they complain about the picky eater. There
she sits, toying with her food, on and on for forty minutes while the exasperated mother could be doing other
things. Today, the neat, tidy eater is on a diet. The picky
eater is still a picky eater—and slender.

AND NEVER SERVE FINGER FOOD

Teaching yourself to eat more slowly isn't easy, but once you recognize the necessity, you can find ways. Prove to yourself that a little food spread over a long time can be quite filling. Never employ a soup spoon. Put away the dinner forks and make do with the salad fork. Even then, try to make a habit of spearing the fork only half full. Half-full teaspoons, too. Eat an entire meal with the aid of a junior-size set of utensils—not the little baby-size silver ones but the in-between size with the dull knife designed to protect children from cutting themselves. Or use a demitasse spoon and your smallest cocktail fork. The little spoon probably won't make it through the consommé, and a good-sized salad will take forever to finish. You'll feel stuffed before dessert.

5. DECALORIZE. I borrowed the term "decalorize" from my friend Ruth West, who coined it in her splendid trend-setting cookbook, *Stop Dieting, Start Losing.* Ruth postulated that all your favorite recipes can remain intact as you craftily replace many high-calorie ingredients with low-calorie equivalents. Proceed in easy, sneaky steps over the months. By the time you've prepared and revised the dish ten or twelve times, nobody has noticed or kept track of the subtle change.

Most families have collected some treasured recipes they depend upon over and over. Write out your mainstay recipes even though you know them by heart. Then whenever you prepare one of them shave off 2 or 3 percent of the calories. Write down the amount you squeezed out.

Take spaghetti and meatballs as an example: Remove six strands of spaghetti and put six more mushrooms into the sauce. Next time, subtract six more strands and add a little eggplant with the mushrooms. The time after that, steal six more strands and increase the tomato. Soon your family will be dining contentedly on five or six ounces of spaghetti instead of eight.

Do the same thing with the meatballs. Instead of red meat only (four times the cholesterol, two to four times the calories, only half the protein of fish, chicken, veal, or cheese), introduce ground turkey, beans, or a soybean meat substitute. Then pad with a little more chopped onion, some chopped parsley, and a bit of grated carrot. On the day the meatball falls apart, you'll know you've gone too far. Backtrack, eliminating some of the carrot.

The same principle can be applied to all your favorite foods. It's especially effective for desserts, which can do nicely with 20 to 40 percent less sugar. Substitute fresh orange or other sweet fruit juice or purée for the sugar in that favorite cake. Work gradually. The sweet tooth can be weaned if you're patient.

The fact is that many people now are decalorizing without realizing it. Today, if you're serving ice cream and fruit, you'll probably pop a dollop of ice cream atop the fruit. A few years ago, there would have been a dab of fruit atop a mound of ice cream.

To get you started on your own system of decalorizing your favorite dishes, this chart suggests some lower-calorie substitutes for high-calorie standbys. (Calorie counts are given in parentheses.)

TRADITIONAL FOOD	CALORIE-SAVING FOOD	CAL- ORIES SAVED
Apple pie, ⅐ wedge of pie (350)	Baked apple (195)	155
Bagel, 1 (165)	Rye toast, 1 slice (60)	105
Beef, chuck, 4 ounces lean meat (180)	Beef round, 4 ounces lean meat (150)	30
Cheese, American, 1 ounce (105)	Mozzarella, 1 ounce (80)	25
Chicken, fried, 4 ounces (235)	Chicken, broiled, 4 ounces (150)	85
Chocolate cake, frosted, 1/16 of cake (235)	Pound cake, ½-inch slice (140)	95
Chocolate pudding, ½ cup (190)	Chocolate junket, ½ cup (120)	70

TRADITIONAL FOOD	CALORIE-SAVING FOOD	CALORIES SAVED
Clam chowder, New England 1 cup (150)	Clam chowder, Manhattan, 1 cup (75)	75
Corn Muffin, 1 medium (130)	Refrigerator biscuit, 1 (80)	50
Cream, light, 1 tablespoon (30)	Half-and-Half, 1 tablespoon (20)	10
Cream of chicken soup, 1 cup (170)	Chicken noodle soup, 1 cup (65)	105
Egg, fried, 1 (110)	Egg, poached, soft- or hard-cooked, 1 (80)	30
English muffin, 1 (145)	Toast, 2 slices (120)	25
Fruit cocktail, canned, ½ cup (95)	Fruit salad, un- sweetened refrig- erated, ½ cup (55)	40
Grapefruit juice, sweetened, 1 cup (130)	Grapefruit juice, unsweetened 1 cup (100)	30
Ice cream, 16% butterfat, 1 cup (375)	Ice cream, 10% butterfat, 1 cup (280)	95
Ice cream, 1 cup (280)	Ice milk, 1 cup (200)	80
Mayonnaise, 1 tablespoon (100)	Salad dressing, 1 tablespoon (65)	35
Milk, whole, 8 ounces (160)	Milk, skimmed, 8 ounces (90)	70
Orange juice, ½ cup (55)	Tomato juice, ½ cup (25)	30
Pecan pie, ⅟₇ of pie (490)	Pumpkin pie, ⅟₇ of pie (275)	215
Pineapple, canned 1 slice, 2 table- spoons syrup (90)	Pineapple, canned in juice, 1 slice 2 tablespoons juice (70)	20

TRADITIONAL FOOD	CALORIE-SAVING FOOD	CALORIES SAVED
Potatoes, fried, homemade, 10 pieces (155)	Potatoes, fried from frozen, 10 pieces (125)	30
Potato chips, 10 medium (115)	Popcorn, buttered, 1 cup (40)	75
Pudding, vanilla, from whole milk, 1 cup (275)	Pudding, vanilla, from skimmed milk, 1 cup (205)	70
Quinine water, 8 ounces (85)	Club soda, 8 ounces (0)	85
Ricotta cheese, ½ cup (170)	Cottage cheese, creamed, ½ cup (120)	50
Salad oil (used) in cooking), 1 table-spoon (125)	Butter or margarine (used in cooking), 1 tablespoon (100)	25
Salmon, canned sockeye, 4 ounces (200)	Salmon, canned pink or chum, 4 ounces (160)	40
Strawberry short-cake, 1 serving with whipped cream (465)	Strawberries in dry wine, 1 serving (100)	365
Sweet potatoes, candied, ½ cup (295)	Winter squash, buttered, ½ cup (95)	200
Yogurt, strawberry flavor, 8-ounce container (290)	Yogurt, vanilla flavor, 8-ounce container (220)	70

Food writers in the United States have been according a lot of space to a ''new'' French cuisine that emphasizes clean, lean crispness without all the fattening sauces considered de rigueur by the old Escoffier school of French chefs. A Washington reporter friend who follows such things thinks the French simply are catching on to a style of cookery that we have been practicing in America for some time.

Apparently the French did not change their ways soon enough, for a Paris nutrition conference has leaked the statistics that overeating is killing Frenchmen. It stated that one French person dies every two minutes because of bad eating habits, and during the last quarter century that nation's meat consumption has increased by over 100 percent. The report goes on to say, "Today, in rich countries people no longer die of hunger, but rather of disorders caused by overeating. . . . Although people expend less energy, they have not reduced the size of their meals."

WHY OPT FOR EVEN DECALORIZED POP?

Before we shake our heads over the French, and their fondness for putting a sauce on a sauce, look at our record: U.S. consumption of soft drinks is up 225 percent since 1950.

So-called "soft" drinks are never served at the Golden Door—not even the sugar-free diet kind. Nor will I allow them in my home. I was dismayed to read a survey released by *Advertising Age* which disclosed that Americans are now guzzling more pop than coffee, formerly the number-one beverage. According to the survey, the per capita figure for 1976 was a whopping 34.8 gallons for each of us. Whatever happened to drinking a glass of water when thirsty?

6. STAY AWARE. Look at your plate and learn how to gauge what is on it; correlate it with what you have eaten and what you will eat ("It's lunch now. What did I eat for breakfast, and what will I be having for dinner?"). Before each meal, ask yourself, "What have I already done today, what am I about to do?" Eat accordingly. A day of driving, telephoning, and desk work suggests a light breakfast and luncheon. But if this is the day you're playing four sets of tennis you can say, "Aha! I deserve an extra piece of toast! I've earned it!"

7. HOW TO SURVIVE A COCKTAIL PARTY. One of

the bonuses of new vitality is that you'll be finding time for all the tempting social invitations sent you, and you'll receive more of them. One of the drawbacks is that you'll wend your way again and again to that fattening tribal gathering, the cocktail party.

Before leaving your home, have a healthful snack to raise your blood-sugar level so you won't be too famished when you arrive at the party. Slice yourself a big piece of melon, or prepare a dish of strawberries or a salad. If you're short of time, take along some sliced raw vegetables to nibble in the car.

If the invitation reads six-thirty, make your entrance at seven-fifteen. This has nothing to do with fashionable lateness; it's just that by seven-thirty or so the hors d'oeuvres will have been picked over, saving you from tantalizing temptations. Also, you'll have time for no more than two drinks, maximum, before dinner.

Once you've joined the party, if you're anything like me, you should locate the peanuts in order to decide the part of the room you're not going to be in. It's simpler to avoid them. And never station yourself within reach of the hors d'oeuvres or the buffet table. Make certain to be as far from it as you can.

Now for the heart of the matter—the cocktail itself. In Washington, D.C., the cocktail party is absolutely a way of life, so I was startled to hear a friend there say she's managed to switch completely away from hard liquor. "I haven't had a drop for three years because I remember you saying three ounces of wine costs us the same number of calories as an ounce of hard liquor. I never cared much about liquor anyway. The only thing I drink now is wine—usually in the form of a spritzer, because soda water makes it go even farther." This is no longer the exception; it is the rule.

If you don't want to wrench yourself from a lifetime of martinis to one of white-wine spritzers, start weaning yourself by asking for a tall glass of club soda with lime when you arrive at a party. It will quench your thirst. Then have your first alcoholic drink. After that, if you still want something to sip, have another club soda with lime, alternating in this fashion till dinnertime.

THE FINEST
SPARKLING WINE IS
NATURAL EFFERVESCENCE

Where else these days, except at a cocktail party, can you feel free to laugh as freely as you like? For most normally gregarious people, it's the friends and new acquaintances, not the drinks and the snacks, that make any such gathering a stimulating one. You get high on people. Most often the drink in your hand is primarily a versatile prop, a sharing of the spirits. Listen raptly or be a chatty raconteur. A goblet filled with naturally carbonated Perrier water is a timely bit of chic that can make you feel and look just as effervescent as if you were sipping champagne.

THE ESSENCE OF GOOD NUTRITION:
QUALITY IN YOUR FOOD

So far, you've covered just two elements of a three-hundred-sixty-five-day health horoscope: First, how to balance energy intake with energy output (remember, the iron law of calorie control is the same as the First Law of Thermodynamics: a definite amount of heat can be converted into a definite amount of energy) and, second, some very logical ways to augment the sheer satisfaction of eating. The missing third element is, of course, good nutrition.

The next time you look at the "enrichments" and additives listed on a food container (I assume you regard the ingredients statement as required reading), reflect for a moment on what standards you have a right to set for your body's fuel. Ask yourself what was removed from the product to make some of those additives necessary. Think for a moment. And then ask yourself where the preservatives go? You're mistaken if you suppose these chemicals will preserve you.

Barbra Streisand ended a lifelong affair with junk foods during a week at the Golden Door, without anything like the struggle she thought she would endure:

I was so sure I was going to feel deprived that, before I went, I stocked up on hot dogs and Cokes . . . but it was wonderful, and my skin was as clear as a bell. It isn't a radical thing with me—the food there was organic, but it doesn't have to be. . . . Just eat good healthful food. The point is, if you know that what you're putting into your system is good, it makes you feel good about yourself.

Food processing and packaging constitute the largest industry in our country. The amount of this production that qualifies as junk food or fast food or convenience food, and the amounts spent in their promotion, run into astronomical figures. We're bogged in $1.5 billion in potato chips alone.

MEET THE GREAT IMPOSTORS OF THE PACKAGED-FOOD INDUSTRY

ACIDULANTS (ACIDS, ALKALIES, BUFFERS, AND NEUTRALIZING AGENTS). To keep soft drinks, processed cheeses, and sherbets from being too tart or too sour.

ANTICAKING AGENTS. To keep salt and powders free-flowing.

BLEACHES AND MATURING AGENTS. To whiten flour and to bleach other products such as cheeses.

CLARIFYING AGENTS. To remove particles which cloud liquids.

COLORS. Over 90 percent are synthetic—most of them coal-tar derivatives. They are insinuated into nearly every imaginable kind of food and drink: meats, wines, margarines and cheeses, potato chips, soft drinks, cakes, gelatin desserts, breads, fruits, cereals, nuts, and soups. On them you'll note the label "U.S. Certified," which gives the impression of having been certified for safety. Here, "certified" means only that the color has met government standards which guarantee neither safety nor purity, since the standards allow a certain percentage margin for impurities.

CURING AGENTS. Nitrite, for example, which also stabilizes color and may have some preservative effect. Its wide use has been linked to cancer.

EMULSIFIERS, STABILIZERS, AND THICKENERS. To make cream seem thick; keep oil and water from separating in margarine; keep oil and vinegar from separating in salad dressings; and give that almost plastic-looking smooth, uniform texture to bread, bakery products, and ice cream.

FIRMING AGENTS. To keep processed fruits from softening.

FLAVOR-ENHANCERS. MSG (monosodium glutamate, or "Accent"), disodium guanylate, maltol and ethyl maltol, and inosinate bring out flavors in foods so that manufacturers are able to add smaller amounts of real ingredients for flavoring. (Synthetic fruit flavors such as strawberry and wintergreen serve the same dubious purpose.)

FOAMING AGENTS AND FOAM INHIBITORS. To make soft drinks bubble. Or to keep them from bubbling too much.

HUMECTANTS. To keep moisture in certain foods—coconut and marshmallows, for example.

NONNUTRITIVE SWEETENERS. Principally saccharin, since cyclamen was banned in 1970. Saccharin, as you know, is on shaky ground. Warming up in the wings, we're told, is the new substitute called Aspartame.

NUTRIENTS. Vitamins and minerals used to "enrich" or "fortify" food staples (such as bread, rice, and potatoes) which during processing were stripped of so many natural nutrients.

Sweden derives 42 percent of its dietary iron (routinely added to "enriched" flours in both our countries) from fortified foods. Swedish doctors are now disturbed because this iron overload can trigger a sometimes fatal hereditary disease. And at Scripps Clinic and Research Foundation in La Jolla, California, hematologist William Crosby has issued a warning against the U.S. proposal to triple the iron which "enriches" our flour and breads.

PRESERVATIVES AND ANTIOXIDANTS. To keep meat from changing color, bread from molding, fruits from turning brown, and fats from tasting and smelling rancid. The best known and most widely used are BHA (butylated hydroxanisole) and BHT (butylated hydroxytoluene). Also calcium disodium EDTA. Such preservatives increase a product's shelf life. They eliminate the need for refrigeration, and for the frequent shipping which used to ensure fresher products.

SEQUESTRANTS. To keep beverages from clouding.
All add their cumulative burdens to our already overworked digestive systems.

ALL STRUNG OUT ON CHAIN FOOD

With almost 50 percent of U.S. mothers working, the massive multimillion-dollar sales campaigns pushing manufactured food products find a large, susceptible market, whether for the frozen TV dinner or the quick-food chain. As Marian Burros, author of the fine book *Pure and Simple,* says, Americans eat one out of every five meals in "some sort of restaurant."

It's estimated that, by 1985, Americans will eat one out of every two meals away from home. Presumably, most of the business will go to the chain restaurants, and bulk preparation and preservation will isolate us from the good health to be found in simple, natural foods.

OUR CANDY KIDS

All along I too have been a working mother. And I know it takes sustained effort to find a workable solution. But when I contemplate the problem of what children are being offered to eat away from home and in the school cafeterias, I am sure that only an enormous education program can save our kids from being junkfood junkies. One small Maryland experiment in exposing preschool children to a variety of delicious and healthful foods seems nearly obliterated by the national sales figures of one breakfast cereal called Cookie Crisp.

Deplorably, the junk-food ban in schools, which Congress was empowered to invoke a year ago, now is bogged down in hearings and cannot possibly be enforced before Autumn 1979.

MOTHER NEEDS A CRASH COURSE IN INVESTIGATIVE REPORTING

While the kids are being bombarded psychologically, their hard-pressed mothers virtually have to subscribe to a clipping service in order to keep up with safe, desirable child nutrition.

Mother has to cope with saturation advertising, and be on the leading edge of such questions as which are the four principal breakfast cereals containing more than 47 percent sugar (probably Cocoa Pebbles, Fruity Pebbles, Honeycomb, and Kellogg's Apple Jacks).

Previously Mother only had to worry about the junkiness of hamburgers, and what percentage of the hamburger was actually meat. Now she has to be alert for hamburgers that might have been cooked at temperatures above 300° F. (suspected of producing cancer-related substances).

WAYS TO ENSURE QUALITY IN YOUR FOOD

1. Eat the freshest fruits and vegetables;
   if possible, grow a small garden.
2. Select the most natural unprocessed foods
   (those without additives or preservatives).
3. Don't listen to fibs about fibre.

4. Understand cholesterol, the chancy fat: There's a little good and a little bad in everybody.
5. Avoid excess sugar, and recognize it in all its deceitful disguises.
6. Really pinch on salt; more and more, learn how to substitute tasteful herbs.
7. Look to the quality of water.

1. THE FRESHEST FRUITS AND VEGETABLES. I once read a U.S. Department of Agriculture pamphlet that traced the vitamin C content of a head of lettuce traveling from field to market to restaurant. This particular head lost 85 percent of its vitamin C before it reached a salad bowl. Food on most family tables is not fresh. Oddly enough, the offender here isn't The System—it's the American housewife.

Here's what happens in many cities. That head of lettuce is picked and rushed to a nearby packinghouse where the outer leaves are removed; the lettuce is washed, crated, and flung onto a truck. That very night the truck rushes down the highway and arrives in a produce market at two in the morning. At four, your local supermarket picks up the lettuce and at six a shift goes on to set out the fresh produce.

Later that day the efficient American housewife drops by with her weekly shopping list. It says she needs three heads of lettuce. Into her shopping cart they go, to languish in her refrigerator for many days. Also on her list are string beans and carrots. In they go with her weekly purchases, although the green string beans look yellow and limp, and she could have taken home fresh, sleek, shiny eggplant.

Ideally, we all should live by Confucius' dictum about diet: Eat nothing but fresh food, in season, locally grown. Obviously, we can't. But 80 percent out of a hundred wouldn't be bad. In the average supermarket you're offered numerous choices. Treat yourself to nothing but the best foodstuffs. You will find them more affordable once you begin to shop every day and for the exact number of people you will be feeding, as well as the appropriate amount each person requires.

LIFE-ENHANCING FOODS
COME ON STRONG

Select foods that stir your senses. Shop with eyes and tactile senses alert for the most bedazzling colors, scents, and textures. It's one way to determine how close your food is to its natural state, straight out of the earth or off a tree. Food which provides this kind of sensory satisfaction has a better chance of providing the Total Calorie all of us need.

Once I visited Paris when the children were small, and because I wanted babysitters we stayed at a little pension-like hotel. There was no menu choice. We ate what was put before us. Since we usually lunched at different restaurants, I would ask the cook what she planned for dinner so we wouldn't eat the same thing two meals in a row. On the third day she slammed down a pot, whirled on me with her arms waving, and screamed, "How can I know what will leap into my market basket?"

She shopped daily—with an empty basket, an almost-empty purse, and an open mind. She bought what was in season, freshest, and best. So should we.

2. SELECT THE MOST NATURAL FOODS. Always remember that we, too, are part of nature; we do best with that which is closest to nature. I'm not advocating moving to a cabbage patch, but I'm a great believer in home gardens, whenever and wherever possible. The advantages stretch beyond the realm of nutrition and touch on every aspect of the Total Calorie.

Puttering in a vegetable garden is one of the finest of exercises. Physically, it provides caloric expenditure and a vast array of sensory diversions. Psychologically, it can transform the most meager salad into an object of infinite pride and satisfaction.

Another bell-ringing bonus, home-grown or not: fresh fruits and vegetables require minimal cooking time. Just add a bit of water or a few lettuce leaves to them in a tightly sealed, heavy pan (not aluminum). No need for sauces or strong seasonings, which only interfere with texture and color.

Simplicity is the keynote. There's a world of difference between a teaspoon of cornflakes and a bite out of a fresh ear of corn. Beware of processing, which in food means to add, subtract, modify, and transform.

TO MARKET, TO MARKET

To reinforce your new convictions, as you wait at the checkout stand always look closely at the cart in front of you and only then at the person beside it. You will find a direct correlation between the contents of the cart and the person who selected them. The cart loaded with boxes and cans, loaves of white bread and six-packs of pop belongs to the harried-looking, old-for-her-age woman you scarcely notice. Then glance at your own cart and say, "Here is my energy, my family's health."

3. DON'T LISTEN TO FIBS ABOUT FIBRE. Once bran was an inseparable part of the American diet. It nearly disappeared save for warm, yummy bran muffins. Now reinstated as the ultimate fibre, bran has a new image.

I agree with the current emphasis on all fibrous foods. They always have been a precondition to any easy process of peristalsis (contraction by which the intestines force their contents onward). Furthermore, fibrous foods are acclaimed for their ability to hold moisture, the natural lubricant of the intestinal tract. Processed foods, in contrast, induce constipation.

Besides, fibrous foods definitely can give you a "full-up" feeling with fewer calories.

4. UNDERSTAND CHOLESTEROL, THE CHANCY FAT. There's a little good and a little bad in everybody. Cholesterol is a combination of fat and protein, known technically as a lipoprotein. Just now there is lively controversy concerning how we get it and how we can get rid of it. Be on the lookout for the most up-to-date information, then carefully weigh all theories against one another.

There is present agreement about one aspect of the controversy. Science now recognizes that cholesterol comes in two varieties: so-called good-guy, high-den-

sity lipoproteins (HDL) and bad-guy, low-density lipoproteins (LDL). It's only LDL that can befoul the walls of
your arteries with dangerous fatty deposits. A prepon-
derance of HDL can even raise your resistance to a coronary.

HAS YOUR CHOLESTEROL REACHED
THE FAT SATURATION POINT?

If you're not blessed with a heredity factor conferring
a high level of HDL, it is rather generally believed that
you can elevate HDL by following the sort of diet this
book advocates (fresh produce, natural whole grains,
fish, not too much meat, not too many dairy products,
and no whole-fat-saturated junk foods). Many experts
think that such a diet plus exercise and weight loss will
encourage your HDL. And an English study further suggests that plenty of vitamin C also might give you an
assist.

THINGS LOOK BLACK FOR
THE LITTLE RED HEN

The chicken or the egg? Many barnyard upsets have
occurred since all-out cholesterol explorations began
anew. Five separate studies, three in the U.S. and two
in central Europe, have tended to exonerate the egg. On
the other hand, Professor Emeritus Raymond Reiser of
Texas A & M insists that chicken is not as utterly blame-
less as we were once told. Cholesterol is in the meat's
membrane, he says, and just as much lurks in chicken
as in beef.

Certain it is that commercially raised and marketed
chickens are on the average a lot fatter than they used
to be. It's been confirmed by research chemists in the
poultry division of the Agricultural Research Service at
USDA.

Despite the poor quality of eggs manufactured in the
modern chicken pen(itentiary), I don't like any of the

egg substitutes. Read the list of their ingredients, and you'll understand why. Don't shy away from eggs and cheeses and oils entirely. If your physician recommends caution, whip up omelettes or soufflés using one egg yolk to two egg whites. Look for some of the fine skim-milk and semi-skim-milk cheeses, and allow yourself two or three of those for each one of the whole-milk variety.

A PRO DEBUNKS THE HIGH-PROTEIN DIET CRAZE

Make your meals from as great a variety of natural foodstuffs as possible. A very pleasant week of simple dinner menus could be constructed around fish twice, chicken once, cheese and/or egg dish twice, and vegetable/proteins twice (consult an inexpensive paperback, *Diet for a Small Planet,* for specific charts clearly outlining the best combinations for converting vegetable proteins into dynamite complete protein).

Remember not to overdo on protein. Many physicians deplore the high-protein diet. Some athletes have self-prescribed excessively high protein in the expectation that it will improve their performance. Dr. Herman Johnson, acting chief, division of bioenergetics, Letterman Institute of Research, San Francisco, debunks this as one of the oldest myths in sports. Many non-athletes have put themselves on a similar diet, under the mistaken impression that, because over-refined sugar and flour are *verboten,* all carbohydrates should be avoided; and in the belief that all proteins are good, and one can't get too much of a good thing.

Excess protein, which cannot be stored as such in the body, has surprised many amateur theorists by turning into fat, just as excess sugar and flour would.

OIL, A SLIPPERY SUBJECT

Eat 100 percent polyunsaturated oils, until there's 100 percent evidence that it's wise to do otherwise. But don't use oil lavishly even if it is polyunsaturated.

Bear in mind that originally most salad-dressing recipes were circulated by salad-oil companies. That's why they usually call for equal parts oil and vinegar. Give the edge to the vinegar. I prefer to dilute the required oil with lemon juice, yogurt, low-fat cheese, tomato juice, or even water. You'll like the taste just as well. Confine yourself to sesame, safflower, and corn oil. If you are extremely fond of olive oil, as I am, then blend one-half olive with one-half corn oil when preparing salads, keeping in mind that 42 percent of the national diet is fat and that the U.S. Government recommends reducing the percentage to 30 percent fat.

Although not all physicians and scientists are in agreement about cholesterol, the consensus is reflected in the above advice. But don't forget that exercise and intelligent weight loss are as integral to good health as is a balanced menu.

5. AVOID EXCESS SUGAR, and recognize it in all its deceitful forms. To me, two of the most depressing sets of annual statistics are those concerning U.S. consumption of refined sugar and soft drinks.

Many researchers are beginning to look critically at that box of sugar on your shelf. It's under suspicion as a possible cause of many of today's diseases. One of the first to sound the alarm was Dr. John Yudkin, formerly professor of nutrition at the University of London. Some of the points he has made:

1. Refined sugar is a poison in the doses many people take of it.

2. The old adage that sugar gives you more energy than other foods is phony. Energy is another word for calories, and you get them from any food.

3. Natural sugar, from raw fruits and unprocessed vegetables, is perfectly all right. You can't eat enough to overdose on it, since it's in combination with its host fruit, which contains all the proper proportions of minerals, vitamins, and enzymes.

WHY ARE ONE-FOURTH
OF YOUR CALORIES EMPTY?

The sad fact is that Americans get only 3 percent of their sugar from fruits and vegetables but sugar represents 24 percent of the calories they consume.

The confections known as packaged breakfast cereals, and the way in which they have been hawked to children via TV commercials, have aroused protests. During nine months of 1975, U.S. children were exposed to only four TV ads for meat, milk, cheeses, or vegetables while they were barraged with 4,000 commercials for sugary products.

SECRET SUGAR,
SURREPTITIOUS SYRUP, ET AL.

Secret sugar, many experts have suspected, constitutes an even greater health threat. March 1978 *Consumer Reports* revealed this to be all too true. Wishbone Russian Dressing, by report of the magazine's celebrated lab, conceals three times as much sugar as Coca-Cola contains. Heinz Tomato Ketchup harbors more sugar than you'll find in most of the popular brands of ice cream. Coffee-mate Non-dairy Creamer has 65 percent, to 51 percent in a milk-chocolate Hershey bar. You'll agree that these revelations are flabbergasting.

It appears that Ritz Crackers are only masquerading—with 12 percent sugar, they would seem to belong in the cookie section. Despite its disarming name, Quaker 100% Natural Cereal is 23.9 percent sugar. Hamburger Helper, nearly one-quarter sugar, offers the kind of help that hamburger doesn't need. The magazine article did not take into account frozen foods, but if you are into seriously checking lists of contents as everyone should be, you must realize that it's difficult to buy a pouch of sugarless green beans. Or peas. Or carrots.

To sum it all up, I again quote *Consumer Reports:* Last year each person in the U.S. averaged 128 pounds of sugar, 14 percent more than seventeen years ago.

Do you truly enjoy your food 14 percent more than you did in 1960? Not if you have total recall of what food used to taste like.

6. AVOID EXCESS SALT. Really pinch on salt. According to metabolic studies, most people require no more than one-tenth of a teaspoon of salt daily. More and more, learn how to substitute tasteful herbs. Excess salt, like sugar, is bad for you. Its effects are cumulative, and as little as three grams a day (about one teaspoon) will contribute to hypertension.

Learn finesse in the use of seasonings like herbs and spices, and puréed vegetables and fruits. All can be imaginative, satisfying substitutes.

The other day I tried some oregano on popcorn. Good. Popcorn is a dandy source of fibre and an all-around good appetite-spoiler if butter/margarine/oil and salt don't ruin its low-calorie status. I think so highly of popcorn that some years ago at Rancho La Puerta we ground it and used the flour for breading carrot cutlets and the like. So far this year I have sprinkled thyme, cumin, or basil on my unbuttered popcorn as substitute for salt.

Secret salt has become as much of a plague as secret sugar. Sodium-low raw peas after they are canned or frozen often have their salt content increased by 200–300 percent. Now a consumer-advocacy group is petitioning the government to require that manufacturers' labels disclose secret salt.

7. LOOK TO THE QUALITY OF WATER. Pure fresh water is a primary consideration. Your body itself is composed chiefly of water. For both drinking and cooking, obtain good spring water with all trace minerals intact.

Do drink the recommended six to eight glasses of fluid each day, always between meals, never with. You can flavor it with freshly squeezed lemon juice if you wish. Just as I anticipate a shower, when I raise my water glass, I like to picture my insides being washed.

THE PLUS AND MINUS WAY
TO BALANCE YOUR WEIGHT

When I had to come up with a plan to help a busy executive follow a weight-loss program and still accommodate business luncheons, cocktails, and dinner engagements, I created a technique you may find helpful too.

It's a system of balances: pluses and minuses. Starting tomorrow, spend a minute each day grading yourself on the previous day. Enter on your calendar a plus if you ate too much; a minus if you were an angel and ordered yogurt and fruit for lunch and fish and a vegetable for dinner; and a zero for the day you neither lost nor gained.

You'll quickly become very handy at setting up in advance a couple of days of compensatory minuses when you intend to dine well on Friday, Saturday, or Sunday. In the same way you'll become quietly proficient at squeezing in an extra hour of exercise that might balance your food intake.

On Monday, review the week past. If you earn one extra minus a week, you most likely have achieved for yourself a laudable deficit of about 875 calories. Four such weeks a month can mean a loss of one pound of fat.

A man using the system can now join in decision-making in which he was merely a bystander. Contemplating a coming day in which he has a business luncheon and his wife has a board-meeting, he may say to her, "My love, let's a both order cottage cheese and salad for lunch. Then let's have eggplant and fish for dinner tonight—there's no way we can keep tomorrow from being a plus." What is so revolutionary about this simple system—and has made it a watchword among Golden Door guests—is that it involves both partners, many for the first time, in determining what they eat.

You will find it much more pleasurable to eat less the day before a high-food event than to punish yourself the day following by dieting.

KNOW THYSELF. Here is an important perception

that the Golden Door teaches as it modifies your attitudes toward food:

Each time you regard any dish of food set before you, pause a moment, think, say if you like, "This is me, my vitality, my body, the fuel for my day." See the food as units of energy hopping all over the plate—"This part I will use during my exercise, this part for sitting at my desk, this part for sleeping, and oh! do I want to store this or leave it on my plate?"

WHY VEGETARIANISM?

If vegetarianism is your thing, as it is mine, you'll find medical research increasingly supportive.

Macrobiotic vegetarians, checked against people who were quite similar except for being nonvegetarian, show lower blood pressure and leaner bodies. Now a scientific team in Boston has reported that a commune-based vegetarian group, carefully studied and tested, showed significantly lower blood cholesterol and triglyceride levels—important factors associated with lower risk of heart attack.

The research team, from Boston City Hospital and Harvard Medical School, measured the blood lipids, or fats, in 116 vegetarians whose diets consisted of whole grains, beans, fresh vegetables, seaweed, and fermented soy products. For additional foods, the vegetarians like fruits, nuts, beer, and fish. Some eat dairy foods; a few eat eggs. These subjects were matched for age and sex with nonvegetarians on the usual American diet. Blood-fat scores were found strikingly low in the vegetarians, who had only slight rises with increased age. Eating dairy foods and eggs increased the lipid scores; but fish, though eaten more often, had no effect on cholesterol or triglyceride levels.

AS CARNIVORES,
WE HUMANS JUST CAN'T CUT IT

"The dental structure of herbivorous animals consists of sharp cutting incisors, while the molars have a flat or nodular surface used for crushing and grinding food. This presupposes that such animals are phylogenetically constructed to live on vegetables, leaves, roots, fruits, nuts, and berries. . . . Examination of the dental structure of modern man reveals that he possesses all the features of a strictly herbivorous animal.'' So said Dr. W. S. Collens of Maimonides Hospital, Brooklyn, at a medical conference. Commenting on the rising preference for vegetarianism among runners, James Fixx in his *Complete Book of Running* presented two conclusions:

1. Man was never designed to eat meat;
2. Consequently, nature made inadequate provision for man to tolerate cholesterol in foods.

THE VIRTUE-MAKING DAY— BETTER THAN FASTING

Perhaps you're feeling heavy and stale after a party weekend or a long stretch of sedentary work. Maybe you'd like to drop a few pounds. If so, try the Virtue-Making Day (so called by the first guests who ever tried it because it made them feel so saintly), which almost all guests follow for one day at the Door and then take home.

This plan is so much more comforting than a day of fasting; because you have continuous blood-sugar builders, you should feel neither hungry nor weak; and there's no chance of loss of body tissue.

NOTES FOR THE VIRTUE-MAKING DIET

This regimen is recommended for people in average good health but is not advised for those troubled by diabetes, hypoglycemia, or any condition requiring medical care. Do check with your physician if you have any doubts.

1. No to coffee and tea. Yes to freshly squeezed, unsweetened lemonade, herb teas, and spring water—as much and as often as you please.

2. You must consume liquids slowly, using a demitasse spoon. Nibble (just as slowly) on the sunflower seeds, which should be hulled, raw, and unsalted. Chew them one by one, with distinct relish.

3. Before each mini-meal, or juice break, step outdoors, even if it's snowing. Breathe consciously. About twenty times, inhale deeply and exhale very, very slowly and thoroughly. Imagine a total oxygen exchange throughout your mind/body. Remain aware of your mind/body as you return to your day.

You will find this day so much more comfortable and comforting than a day of fasting, because you have continuous blood-sugar builders every two and a half hours—a juice break providing diversion and sustaining resolve. You should feel neither hungry, weak, nor tense.

Our three-meal-a-day habit was made to suit man's convenience, but man was not made to suit the three meals. We are probably most suited to a nutritionally balanced simulation of the Virtue-Making Diet which would approximate the ideal situation of several small and adequate snack/meals: exactly enough to keep blood-sugar and energy level high but not enough to add to the body store of fat. For when early man foraged for food he often could not eat to satiety; with him usually it was feast or famine. That is why our bodies are equipped to accommodate a large meal (and our stomachs stretch as the meal requires) but accept only the energy we need and store the rest away as converted fat (ladies do this better, for they have thirty percent more fat cells than men because of their early need to nourish, first, the child within and then the helpless human baby throughout times of famine).

Today famine no longer plagues us, and how could Mother Nature have anticipated that some day we would be assaulted not by predators competing with us for food but by appetite stimuli like the TV ads, the overstocked supermarkets, or the overloaded refrigerator.

Like the Virtue-Making Diet, the Golden Door's approximately one-thousand-calorie-a-day regimen keeps high both physical and psychological energy.

And here I reiterate my belief in our total food program with its inclusion of planned midmorning and midafternoon balanced snacks.

DIET FOR
THE GOLDEN DOOR
VIRTUE-MAKING DAY

(Note: with the exception of almond milk, with each serving of liquid eat ½ ounce sunflower seeds and 3 pine nuts.)

8:00 A.M. GRAPEFRUIT JUICE
>   4 oz. freshly squeezed grapefruit juice
>   2 oz. water
>
> Mix and serve.

10:30 A.M. ALMOND MILK
>   6 whole almonds, blanched and peeled
>   ½ medium-sized ripe banana
>   ½ cup water
>   2 ice cubes
>   few drops fresh lemon juice
>   dash of vanilla
>   dash of nutmeg
>
> Place in blender, liquefy, and serve.

1:00 P.M. GAZPACHO
>   1 medium tomato, peeled and diced
>   ¼ large cucumber, peeled and chopped
>   ¼ large green pepper, seeded and chopped
>   1 onion slice
>   2 sprigs parsley
>
> Place in blender, liquefy, and serve.

3:30 P.M. PINEAPPLE-CUCUMBER JUICE
>   3 oz. cucumber, peeled
>   1 oz. fresh pineapple
>   2 sprigs parsley
>   2 oz. apple juice
>
> Place in blender, liquefy, and serve.

6:00 P.M. ALMOND MILK

8:30 P.M. CARROT-APPLE JUICE
          2 oz. apple juice
          2 oz. carrot juice
          ⅓ apple, peeled
          Place in blender, liquefy, and serve.

HERBEVERAGES

As an alternate to the more universal appetite-spoilers and cooling beverages, the Golden Door introduces to its guests the novelty of fresh fruit juices combined with herbal teas. The one fortifies the other. Many well-known beneficial herbs have a pleasant and distinctive taste. When blended with juice they produce original low-calorie flavors which are nutritious alternatives to bottled soft drinks.

Here are a few herbeverages created at the Golden Door. The concept is still so new that you may wish to experiment further as different fruits come into season:

PINK MINT TEA

3 cups pink mint tea   dab of honey
1 cup unsweetened
   grape juice

Combine all ingredients, chill well, pour into a pre-chilled thermos—approximately 42 calories per serving. (Serves 6)

CRANBERRY HERB TEA

3 cups camomile tea   dab of honey
1 cup unsweetened
   cranberry juice

Combine all ingredients, chill well, pour into a pre-chilled thermos—approximately 42 calories per serving. (Serves 6)

RED CLOVER HIBISCUS TEA

3 cups red clover tea
brewed with one
cup hibiscus tea

1 cup pear juice
honey to taste

Combine all ingredients, chill well, pour into a pre-chilled thermos—approximately 35 calories per serving. (Serves 6)

PINK LEMON TEA

3 cups pink-lemon
herb tea
1 cup strawberry or
other berry juice

dab of honey

Combine all ingredients, chill well, pour into a pre-chilled thermos—approximately 20 calories per serving. (Serves 6)

TROPICAL TEA

3 cups pink mint tea
1 cup coconut milk

few drops banana
extract

Combine all ingredients, chill well, pour into a pre-chilled thermos—approximately 25 calories per serving. (Serves 6)

ROSE APPLE TEA

2 cups rose hip tea
2 cups apple juice

dash cinnamon

Combine all ingredients, chill well, pour into prepared thermos—approximately 58 calories per serving. (Serves 6)

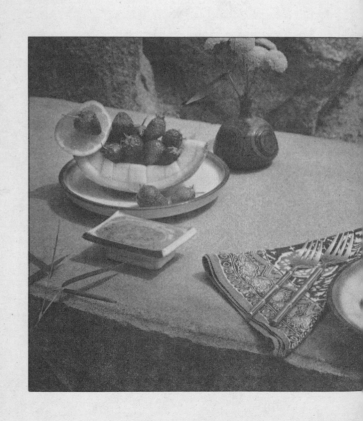

CHAPTER IX

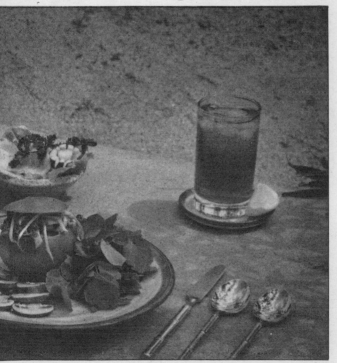

THE GOLDEN DOOR
MENUS AND RECIPES

INTRODUCING THE
GOLDEN DOOR MENUS

Years ago, I spent many exhausting hours in the kitchen at Rancho La Puerta preparing meals for our early guests. Daily I ground wheat, baked bread, milked goats and made cheese, rinsed sprouts, nursed our acidophilus-milk culture, and grew, canned, and cooked in the sun a great assortment of vegetables and fruits.

My guests of today are being served with every bit as much pride, but far less effort. The superb and simple Golden Door food, in the opinion of many, is my spa's most outstanding claim to fame. It anticipated by many years the *cuisine minceur* of present-day French chefs.

Now my time in food preparation has been reduced to an occasional precious and privileged hour in my own kitchen on a quiet Sunday. But in my fancy I never really have left the kitchen. I still frequent the delicious territory of my cookbook shelf—I feel that if a recipe cannot in itself arouse my taste buds, it isn't worth cooking.

The following menus and recipes are selected from the hundreds of favorites served at the Golden Door. They represent one full month—four weeks of tantalizing, satisfying food, planned to help you normalize your weight. As you turn the pages, try to smell, savor, and visualize each dish. They are all the more delectable because almost every ingredient is fresh and unprocessed.

In assembling the menus and recipes, I've tried to create an eating plan that can gracefully be adapted to many life-styles. I've chosen menus that will fit easily into your eating patterns—meals that are varied, quick, and enjoyable to prepare, yet satisfying at your dinner table.

It would be preposterous to try to create the perfect diet for the average person. There is no perfect diet. And, as I have said before, there is no average person. Use the following meals and recipes as a loose frame for you to adjust and readjust around the shifting elements of your everyday life.

Each recipe is low in calories, but all calorie counts are necessarily approximate—for the size and even the quality of an ingredient will affect the total calorie content.

There are twenty-eight menus in all; four groups of seven each compose a hypothetical week. In each group, five of the menus are arranged as dinners for two. If you are cooking for more than two who wish to lose weight, you can easily multiply the ingredients. Each week of menus also contains a low-calorie entertainment dinner for six. Completing the selection is a brunch or late, light supper. Most of the meals can be prepared in thirty to forty minutes, with the exception of the international and entertainment recipes, which you should be able to put together in about an hour.

LOW CALORIE, LOW SODIUM, LOW CHOLESTEROL

The dressings and sauces all were developed at the Golden Door and are significantly reduced in calories. They can be prepared ahead and refrigerated or frozen in small portions to be used as required in many of the recipes. You will note that little or no salt is used in these sauces. Almost all Americans salt their food much too heavily, and for that reason I recommend going light on salt, heavy on herbs and spices—with an ever-vigilant emphasis on fresh ingredients which have undergone the least possible amount of processing. If your doctor has recommended a salt-free diet, increase the herbs and spices and eliminate salt entirely.

A new habit you will wish to acquire—use nature's own fructose as a fine substitute for sugar. Soak a small amount of dried fruit overnight in just enough hot water to cover. In the morning pit and liquefy. Then use the sweet syrup in recipes, over pancakes, and as a fruit-salad topping.

Other alternates: finely chop dates, or stew fruit in fruit juices. For example, stew an apple and a banana in a small amount of apple juice with two or three fine slices of candied ginger—the variations are infinite.

An instant sauce or dressing can be made by blending a piece of cooked vegetable with the juices in which it was cooked and adding a few simple herbs as seasoning. An elegant dessert can be concocted from a slice of really ripe fruit served in a pretty dish and topped with another liquefied fruit of contrasting flavor and color.

The only special equipment you will need is a food blender (liquefier). If you are short on time, you will discover that the Cuisinart, or one of its competitors, does so much more than blend or chop or liquefy; it is an extraordinary substitute for one more pair of hands.

I have not included recipes for breakfast or luncheon. Please see pages 264–65 for suggestions and for the vital discussion of caloric apportionment.

The best way to utilize these menus effectively is to

choose the one that matches your caloric need for the day. For instance, if you overeat at luncheon, choose the dinner menu with the lowest calorie count. The five varied dinner menus for two offer you many options: one is very low-calorie, one is vegetarian, one is international, one is Golden Door gourmet, and one is a quickie, for when you are in a hurry to get on with your evening.

Weight loss should be sensible, steady, and slow, so that vitality will be enhanced and in no way diminished.

If one serving is not sufficient because you have a greater caloric need, there are several alternatives: increase the portion size; add a slice of Tecate Bread (page 384) or a starch such as a potato; include a serving of whole grains like bulgur wheat, brown rice, or buckwheat groats. Spread your Tecate Bread with apple butter, which has fewer calories than butter and still less if homemade without sugar. Do take an afternoon pick-me-up (snack), a wedge of cheese or some nuts and a piece of fruit. Eat more at breakfast and/or luncheon. And remember that portion size should never be dictated by dollars and cents but according to the pounds and inches of the person being served.

Above all, bear in mind that the most important ingredient you can add to a meal is joy. (And, before you turn to the menus and recipes, I want to express thanks for the joyous contribution of Michel Stroot, the best chef the Golden Door has ever had.)

WEEK I
OF DINNER MENUS
FOR WEIGHT REDUCTION

		CALORIES
1	WATERCRESS SALAD	60
Very low cal	MUSHROOM SOUFFLÉ	265
	BANANA-ORANGE CRUNCH	180
	TOTAL:	505

		CALORIES
2	GARDEN SOUP	55
Vegetarian	EGGPLANT PARMESAN	435
	FRUTTO VINO	115
	TOTAL:	605

3	MIDDLE-EASTERN	
International	ANISE BREW	75
	WORRY-BEAD APPETIZER	
	FISH KEBABS	250
	SHREDDED VEGETABLE	
	SALAD	115
	BROILED GRAPEFRUIT	65
	TOTAL:	505

4	OLIVE-STUFFED	
Golden Door	ARTICHOKES	25
Gourmet	CHICKEN CHASSEUR	220
	ZUCCHINI FORMAGGIO	195
	NAVEL ORANGE	75
	TOTAL:	515

5	1 SLICE TECATE BREAD,	
Quickie	TOASTED	100
	TURKEY SALAD DIVAN	270
	CARAMEL CUSTARD	205
	TOTAL:	575

6	ZUCCHINI SALAD	
Brunch or late,	ANDALOUSE	50
late supper	PAUPIETTE OF VEAL	
	ROULATINE	400
	CREAM OF MANGO	
	AU KIWI	100
	TOTAL:	550

7	WHITE-WINE SPRITZER	45
Dinner for six	PEASANT CAVIAR	85
	GOLDEN DOOR	
	BREAST OF CHICKEN	310
	GARDEN OF VEGETABLES	110
	APPIAN PEARS	175
	TOTAL:	725

WATERCRESS SALAD

(Each serving, 60 calories)

The quality of this salad depends on the absolute freshness of the watercress. Spinach and curly endive, mixed half and half, may be substituted if watercress is not available.

½ large tomato, peeled and diced

¼ teaspoon Golden Door seasoning salt (see page 381)

¼ teaspoon freshly ground pepper

1 tablespoon Golden Door vinaigrette dressing (see

dressing for Golden Door Combination Salad, page 341)

1 bunch watercress

1 to 2 ounces fresh bean sprouts

1 teaspoon chopped chives or scallions

1 tablespoon sunflower seeds

Season the tomato and pour the dressing over it. Wash the watercress and remove the stems. Just before serving, add the bean sprouts to the tomato and watercress. Sprinkle with chives and toss. Add the sunflower seeds and toss again. Serve immediately.

MUSHROOM SOUFFLÉ

(Each serving, 265 calories)

1 tablespoon plus 1 teaspoon 100% corn-oil margarine

2 cups finely chopped fresh mushrooms (about ⅓ pound)

¼ cup finely chopped mild onion (Bermuda or green onion, or shallot)

1 very small clove garlic, minced

4 teaspoons unbleached flour

salt, pepper, and nutmeg

2 teaspoons lemon juice

2 tablespoons white wine, milk, or water

3 eggs, at room temperature, separated

Melt 1 tablespoon margarine in frying pan over high heat. Add mushrooms, onion, and garlic. Cook, stirring, until mixture begins to brown and most of the moisture has gone. Remove from heat. Sprinkle with flour, ¼ teaspoon salt, pepper, and a dash of nutmeg. Stir to coat evenly. Add lemon juice and wine, cool, then blend in egg yolks.

Preheat oven to 375° F. Grease 2 soufflé dishes of 1½- to 2-cup capacity with as little margarine as possible.

Beat egg whites with ⅛ teaspoon salt until they hold peaks but still look moist. Fold (don't stir) half the whites into mushrooms until fully blended. Partially fold in remaining whites. Immediately pour into dishes and bake about 15 to 18 minutes, or until centers no longer feel liquid when gently touched. Eat at once. (A soufflé falls less rapidly if served on hot plates and spooned from the outside, not the center.)

BANANA-ORANGE CRUNCH

(Each serving, 180 calories)

1 medium banana, peeled and sliced	2 tablespoons fine graham-cracker crumbs
¼ cup fresh or canned mandarin oranges, drained	1 tablespoon chopped nuts
1 teaspoon honey	1 tablespoon 100% corn-oil margarine
1 teaspoon lemon juice	

Combine banana, oranges, honey, and lemon juice in a bowl and chill. Sauté crumbs and nuts in the margarine over low heat until crumbs are toasted. Place fruit mixture in two dessert dishes and sprinkle with crumbs. *Note:* You may substitute any favorite fruit for the mandarin oranges.

GARDEN SOUP

(Each serving, 55 calories)

- 2 cups chicken broth (see page 383)
- 1 carrot, sliced ¼-inch thick
- 2 green onions, including part of green tops, sliced (reserve remaining green tops)
- ½ cup raw green beans, cut into 1-inch pieces, or broccoli flowerettes
- ½ green or red bell pepper, diced

salt and pepper

Heat chicken broth, add vegetables, and simmer about 5 to 10 minutes, or until vegetables are tender-crisp. About 2 minutes before serving, add reserved green onion tops and season with salt and pepper.

EGGPLANT PARMESAN

(Each serving, 435 calories)

Make the tomato sauce first and then proceed with the recipe. See the recipe for Tomato Sauce (page 382) or use this recipe:

- 1 (8-ounce) can tomato sauce
- 1 large clove garlic, puréed
- ⅛ teaspoon each dried basil and oregano
- ¼ teaspoon anise or fennel seed (optional)

In small saucepan combine all ingredients. Bring to boil and simmer for 20 minutes, stirring occasionally.

4 slices unpeeled
  eggplant, ½-inch
  thick
½ cup nonfat milk
2 tablespoons
  unbleached flour
1 egg
1 tablespoon water
1 green onion with
  part of green top,
  minced
1 tablespoon minced

  fresh parsley
salt and pepper
2 tablespoons olive oil
  (approximate)
2 ounces Swiss or
  Monterey Jack
  cheese, cut into 2
  slices
sprinkle of grated
  Parmesan cheese
tomato sauce

Salt eggplant, marinate in milk for 10 minutes, remove, and pat dry (discard milk).

Put flour on a plate. In bowl wide enough to hold eggplant, blend egg, water, green onion, parsley, salt and pepper to taste. Heat 1 tablespoon oil in large frying pan over medium heat.

Dip each eggplant slice in flour to coat, then in egg mixture. Fry slowly until golden brown. Turn, adding rest of oil to brown other side. Eggplant should be nearly tender when finished. Cool slightly.

Place 1 slice eggplant and 1 slice cheese into individual baking dishes. Top with a second eggplant slice. Smother each with tomato sauce and top with grated Parmesan cheese.

Bake at 375° F. until hot and bubbly (15 minutes if all ingredients are warm when assembled).

FRUTTO VINO

(Each serving, 115 calories)

⅓ cup sherry   1 apple
1 orange

Heat wine just until it starts to simmer, to reduce alcoholic calories. Cool.

Peel orange; remove as much white membrane as possible; slice thinly and remove seeds. Core unpeeled apple, slice thinly, and coat with some juice from the orange to prevent discoloration. Pour wine over fruit and chill, turning once to marinate, about 15 minutes. Serve with slices arranged alternately in bowl with marinade.

INTERNATIONAL

MIDDLE-EASTERN ANISE BREW

(Each serving, 75 calories)

The favorite alcoholic drink all over the Near and Middle East is a clear anise-flavored brew that turns milky when water or ice is added. The Greeks call it ouzo; the Turks, raki; and the Arabs, arrack. This recipe duplicates the flavor.

¼	teaspoon anise extract		wine
		6	ice cubes, cracked
¼	cup very dry white		or crushed

Add extract to wine and stir. Serve over cracked ice.

WORRY-BEAD APPETIZER

Throughout the Middle East, people finger strings of "worry beads" to relieve tension. Unfortunately, it is possible to fiddle with the beads single-handedly, leaving the other hand free for food, drink, and nicotine.

Cracking *unshelled* sunflower seeds, also a Middle Eastern pastime, serves the purpose better than beads. It occupies both hands. Also, the seeds are so tiny and troublesome to get at that it is almost impossible to overeat.

A sunflower-seed researcher armed with calorie-count book, scale, clock, and basic arithmetic produced these startling findings: It took nearly 30 minutes to crack ⅓ cup (or 175 seeds), which weighed ⅓ ounce and had a total calorie count of about 55.

Conclusion: Crack all the sunflower seeds you have patience for, and eat them as an appetizer with your drink before dinner.

FISH KEBABS

(Each serving, 250 calories)

1 tablespoon olive oil
⅔ pound very firm fish, cut into 1-inch cubes

1 lemon
8 bay leaves, broken in half

Sprinkle 1 teaspoon oil over fish. Cut lemon in half and squeeze juice of one half onto fish. Add bay leaves and toss to coat. Marinate for about 15 minutes.

Cut remaining lemon half, including rind, into ¾-inch wedges. Heat remaining 2 teaspoons oil in large frying pan over medium-high heat. Add lemon wedges, cover until spattering dies down, uncover, and sauté until glazed and golden brown. Remove and cool.

Thread 4 to 6 short skewers alternately with fish, lemon wedges, and bay leaves. Broil skewers, turning to brown all sides. Fish is done when no longer translucent inside. Total cooking time should be about 5 to 6 minutes. The charring of bay leaves and lemon is desirable—it contributes delightful flavor.

SHREDDED VEGETABLE SALAD

(Each serving, 115 calories)

The white radish *(beyaz turp)* used in this Turkish salad is the same mild, foot-long type found here in Oriental grocery stores and many supermarkets. Its Japanese name is *daikon;* the Chinese name is *loh bok.*

If you can't find the radish, just make the salad with carrot and cabbage and garnish it with red radishes. Or substitute shredded turnip or raw beet.

lettuce leaves
2 carrots, shredded
1 cup shredded green or red cabbage
1 cup shredded mild white radish

1 tablespoon olive oil
4 pickled peppers *(peperoncino)*
1 lemon, cut into 4 wedges

Line salad plates with lettuce. Toss each shredded vegetable separately with 1 teaspoon oil. On each plate arrange a tricolored mound of the three separate vegetables. Garnish each plate with 2 peppers and 2 lemon wedges. Squeeze lemon juice over salad before eating.

BROILED GRAPEFRUIT

(Each serving, 65 calories)

1 grapefruit, preferably pink	pinch of ground ginger
2 teaspoons brown sugar	2 fresh strawberries, cut in half

Cut grapefruit in half; cut out membrane in center and loosen segments with knife. Sprinkle with sugar and ginger. Place in a baking pan and bake at 375° F. for 15 minutes, or until very hot and bubbly. Put berries in centers. Serve hot.

GOLDEN DOOR GOURMET

OLIVE-STUFFED ARTICHOKES

(Each serving, 25 calories)

If you use fresh cooked artichokes to prepare this, save the leaves with edible tips. Squeeze lemon juice over them and use some for garnish. The rest can be refrigerated for a low-calorie snack or salad.

2 anchovy fillets, minced (optional)	½ teaspoon lemon juice
½ teaspoon drained chopped capers	1 tablespoon minced parsley
2 teaspoons finely chopped black olives	2 cooked artichoke bottoms, coated with lemon juice

Mix anchovies (optional), capers, olives, and lemon juice. Spoon into artichoke cavities. Completely cover with parsley. Chill.

If you have fresh leaves, arrange 12 in a fan shape

around the stuffed artichoke placed at one side of each plate.

Note: The flavor of canned water-packed artichoke bottoms is improved by simmering them in home-made chicken stock before using. Fresh ones should be coated with lemon juice immediately after preparing to prevent discoloration.

CHICKEN CHASSEUR

(Each serving, 220 calories)

1 whole chicken breast, skinned	1 large clove garlic, minced
1 cup chicken broth	6 small mushrooms, sliced
1 cup water	2 small tomatoes, peeled and diced
½ bay leaf	
1 sprig fresh or ½ teaspoon dried thyme	oregano
	¼ teaspoon dried or 1 tablespoon fresh tarragon
⅓ stalk celery	
½ teaspoon Golden Door seasoning salt (see page 381)	⅓ cup dry white wine
	¼ teaspoon minced fresh chives
½ teaspoon olive oil	
½ small onion, chopped	2 teaspoons minced fresh parsley

Cut breast in half and place in saucepan with chicken broth, water, bay leaf, thyme, celery, and salt. Cover and simmer for about 35 minutes, or until breast is ten-der. In the meantime, heat oil in a heavy skillet and add onion and garlic. Sauté until onion is limp. Add mush-rooms and cook for 5 minutes. Add tomatoes, oreg-ano, and tarragon and cook uncovered for about 20 minutes, stirring occasionally, until sauce thickens. Add wine and boil for 10 minutes.

Remove breast from cooking liquid; place each half in a serving dish or individual casserole with a little of the broth in the bottom. Just before serving add chives and parsley to the tomato wine sauce and spoon over chicken.

ZUCCHINI FORMAGGIO

(Each serving, 195 calories)

2 large zucchini,
scrubbed but
unpeeled
2 tablespoons 100%
corn-oil margarine
salt

pepper
2 tablespoons grated
Parmesan cheese
2 tablespoons minced
parsley

Shave tips and stems off zucchini and grate on large holes of grater. Place zucchini in a colander set over a bowl. Let drain for 3 to 4 minutes. Just before cooking, squeeze gently by handfuls. (You may wish to reserve the vegetable juice you squeeze out to add to soups or stews.)

Melt margarine in a skillet. When bubbly, toss in the zucchini and add salt and pepper to taste. Cook until tender-crisp, about 3 to 5 minutes (taste to be sure). Add Parmesan cheese and parsley. Toss together and serve immediately.

QUICKIE

TURKEY SALAD DIVAN

(Each serving, 270 calories)

½ pound fresh broccoli
½ head butter lettuce
2 ounces Gruyère

cheese, thinly sliced
¼ pound turkey, thinly
sliced

Chive Dressing

½ cup plain low-fat
yogurt
2 tablespoons minced
chives
1 tablespoon minced
parsley
2 teaspoons finely
chopped green

onion, including
some of the green
top
salt and pepper
pinch of dried
crumbled tarragon
1 teaspoon Dijon
mustard

In the morning, trim tough ends from the broccoli and split stalks through the flowerettes. Drop into boiling salted water to cover. Bring water back to a boil and cook, uncovered, for 3 to 5 minutes, or until stems can be easily pierced with a fork. Strain, rinse in cold water, and chill.

To make the dressing, mix together all dressing ingredients and chill.

In the evening, when ready to serve, arrange the lettuce, broccoli, cheese, and turkey on platter; pour dressing on top.

CARAMEL CUSTARD

(Each serving, 205 calories)

1 egg	grated peel of ½ lemon
⅔ cup nonfat milk	100% corn-oil
6 teaspoons sugar	margarine

In a mixing bowl, beat egg and blend in milk, 3 teaspoons sugar, and lemon peel, stirring until the sugar dissolves.

Using margarine, grease 2 glass baking dishes or smoothly glazed custard cups of ½-cup size. Set in a baking pan containing 1 inch hot water.

Put 3 teaspoons sugar in heavy saucepan over low heat and stir until sugar melts and begins to brown. Quickly pour into prepared dishes. Cover with the custard mixture.

Bake at 325° F. for about 30 to 35 minutes, until centers no longer jiggle when pressed. Remove from water, cool, and chill.

To serve, loosen around top with knife and dip in hot water a little longer than you would to unmold gelatin. Hold plate over cup, invert quickly, and tap with knife handle or slap with palm to loosen.

ZUCCHINI SALAD ANDALOUSE

(Each serving, 50 calories)

2 medium-sized zucchini

Golden Door seasoning salt (see page 381)

2 large shallots, finely chopped

1 clove garlic, finely chopped

polyunsaturated oil

1 tablespoon chopped chives

¼ teaspoon freshly ground black pepper

¼ teaspoon oregano

1 small red pimiento (fresh, if possible)

dash of cayenne

1 medium-sized tomato

lettuce

parsley

Slice the zucchini into thin rounds, discarding the ends, and season lightly with seasoning salt and cayenne. In a heavy skillet sauté the shallots and garlic in a few drops of oil for a minute or two. Add the zucchini and cook quickly over high heat, stirring. Reduce the heat and cook, covered, for 3 to 4 minutes (zucchini should be slightly crisp). Transfer to a salad bowl and sprinkle with chives. Set aside to cool.

Peel the tomato and dice finely. Season with oregano. Mix well with the zucchini. Remove the core and seeds from the pimiento, dice, and add cayenne. Combine with the zucchini-tomato mixture.

Refrigerate the salad for 2 to 3 hours before serving on a bed of lettuce. Garnish with chopped fresh parsley.

PAUPIETTE OF VEAL ROULATINE

(Each serving, 400 calories)

2 veal scallopinis (about 3½ to 4 ounces each)
freshly ground black pepper
Golden Door seasoning salt (see page 381)
Italian seasoning
¾ pound fresh spinach
dash of nutmeg
½ cup grated Monterey Jack cheese
2 tablespoons freshly grated Parmesan cheese
2 tablespoons freshly toasted pine nuts
1 tablespoon 100% corn-oil margarine
⅛ cup dry white wine
juice of ½ small lemon
10 rigatoni noodles
¼ cup tomato juice
oregano
parsley

Pound the veal thin with the side of a cleaver (or ask the butcher to prepare it for you). Season each scallopini with seasoning salt, pepper, and Italian seasoning. Wash spinach and drain thoroughly. Cook in a tightly covered pan until slightly wilted. Drain thoroughly. Chop spinach coarsely and add seasoning salt, pepper, and nutmeg. In a saucepan combine spinach and Jack cheese. Cook over low heat until the cheese melts. Add the pine nuts and set aside to cool.

Spread each scallopini with half the spinach mixture and roll up, securing with toothpicks. In a heavy casserole brown the scallopini lightly in oil. Cover and bake in a 375° F. oven for 10 minutes. Remove from the oven and add the margarine and white wine. Squeeze the lemon juice over the top. Sprinkle the Parmesan over and return briefly to the oven or under the broiler.

Serve immediately—accompanied by the rigatoni noodles, which have been cooked until tender and then reheated in the tomato juice seasoned with oregano. Garnish the entire dish with parsley.

CREAM OF MANGO AU KIWI

(Each serving, 100 calories)

1 very ripe mango (fresh or canned)	1 tablespoon Grand Marnier
½ cup fresh orange juice	1 firm but ripe kiwi

Peel the mango, remove the stone, and put the pulp into the blender container. Add orange juice and blend for 2 to 3 minutes until creamy. In a small saucepan bring the liqueur to a boil (this removes approximately half the calories). Add the liqueur to the mango and blend again briefly. Divide the mango cream evenly between two dessert dishes. Peel the kiwi, slice into thin rounds, and arrange around the edge of the mango cream. Chill before serving.

DINNER FOR SIX

WHITE-WINE SPRITZER

(Each serving, 45 calories)

⅘ quart dry white wine (Chablis), well chilled	1 quart club soda or sparkling water, well chilled
few dashes Angostura bitters	lemon twists

Pour well-chilled wine into pitcher to half full. Add bitters and club soda. Serve immediately in large wineglasses or in highball glasses, with lemon twists. Makes 12 servings (2 per person).

PEASANT CAVIAR

(Each serving, 85 calories with two crackers)

3 cups eggplant (about 1½ pounds)	onion salt and pepper
2 tablespoons olive oil	6 black olives
1 teaspoon lemon juice	parsley
2 tablespoons minced	12 rye wafers

The night before you plan to serve this appetizer, place the eggplant under the broiler on the lowest rack until the skin becomes charcoal black and eggplant is soft. Be sure to turn it occasionally. When done, peel off the skin without allowing eggplant to cool. Cube the pulp and whirl in the blender until creamy. Measure out 3 cups. Place in a bowl and add oil, lemon juice, onion, and salt and pepper to taste. Whip with a fork until fluffy. Refrigerate.

When ready to serve, garnish with olives and parsley and serve with rye wafers.

GOLDEN DOOR
BREAST OF CHICKEN
(Each serving, 310 calories)

The chicken is stuffed with just a piece of cheese, which melts to look and taste like a rich sauce.

To bone chicken breasts: Bend breast halves until the large bone protrudes so you can pull it out. Use knife to loosen, if necessary. Then insert fingers under membrane with row of little bones; pull all off in one strip.

6 large boneless chicken-breast halves, skinned	1 tablespoon grated Parmesan or Romano cheese
6 strips Monterey Jack or Swiss cheese, each about 3 × 1 × ¼ inches (about ¼ pound)	salt and pepper
	3 tablespoons unbleached flour
3 eggs	2 tablespoons salad or olive oil
1 tablespoon minced parsley	parsley sprigs
	6 lemon wedges

Make a pocket for stuffing each chicken breast by slicing lengthwise from one side partially through. Lay cheese strip inside. Fasten opening with wooden pick; also fasten loose ends into a neat bundle (to be sure no opening remains where cheese may ooze out).

In a bowl, blend eggs, parsley, and grated cheese with salt and pepper to taste. Coat chicken heavily with flour, then roll it completely in the egg mixture.

Heat the oil in small frying pan over medium-high heat. Add chicken with as much egg clinging to it as possible. Spoon remaining egg mixture on top. Fry about 1 minute on each side, just enough to set the coating. (This much can be done ahead of serving time; then refrigerate.)

When ready to serve, place chicken in a baking pan and bake, uncovered, at 375° F. for 25 to 30 minutes, or until coating begins to brown. (If prepared ahead, let come to room temperature before cooking. A few extra minutes' baking may be required.) When you test chicken for doneness, be careful not to puncture where cheese may ooze out.

Remove picks and serve hot with parsley and lemon wedges.

GARDEN OF VEGETABLES

(Each serving, 110 calories)

2½ cups each raw cabbage, broccoli, cauliflower, and green beans (all cut according to instructions in recipe)

2 to 3 tablespoons water

3 tablespoons 100% corn-oil margarine

1 tablespoon salad oil or olive oil

4 cups spinach leaves, cut into 1-inch pieces

salt and pepper

Measure each after cutting: chop cabbage into ½-inch pieces; cut or break broccoli and cauliflower into ½-inch flowerettes; cut beans into ½-inch sections. Put water in saucepan, bring to a simmer, and immediately add all the vegetables *except* spinach. Dribble the oil over, cover, and simmer about 5 minutes—just until vegetables are tender-crisp. Drain in colander.

Put large frying pan or Chinese wok over highest heat, add margarine, and turn pan to coat. Add warm vegetables and spinach all at once. Stir and toss constantly for about 2 minutes while adding salt and pepper to taste, just until vegetables are very hot. Serve at once.

APPIAN PEARS

(Each serving, 175 calories)

3 large pears, peeled, halved, and cored	chopped slivered almonds
¾ cup sherry	½ teaspoon almond extract
6 tablespoons	

Put pears, cored sides up, in smallest possible baking dish. Dribble sherry over. Put almonds and almond extract into cavities. Bake uncovered at 350° F. for 30 minutes, basting with sherry occasionally. Serve hot or cold.

WEEK II
OF DINNER MENUS
FOR WEIGHT REDUCTION

		CALORIES
1	GAZPACHO	70
Very low cal	CHILES RELLEÑOS	
	RANCHO LA PUERTA	230
	TOSTADA SALAD	70
	TECATE SHERBET	125
	TOTAL:	495
2	TOMATO AND CUCUMBER	
Vegetarian	SALAD WITH MUSHROOMS	125
	GARDEN SPAGHETTI	400
	LEMON LIGHTNING	115
	TOTAL:	640
3	*SAKE* MARTINI	50
International	CHICKEN LIVERS YAKITORI	150
	MIZUTAKI FOR TWO	315
	ORANGES IN SNOW	115
	TOTAL:	630
4	CITY GARDEN SALAD	110
Golden Door	FILLET OF SOLE	
Gourmet	IN EGG BATTER	100
	GREEN BEANS STUFATI	100

		CALORIES
	CARROTS CREMATE	110
	FRUIT FOR DESSERT (OR FRUIT AND CHEESE)	210
	TOTAL:	630
5 Quickie	QUICK WELSH RAREBIT	330
	WALDORF SALAD	175
	TOTAL:	505
6 Brunch or late, late supper	VEGETABLES BRAVADO	65
	CHICKEN CACCIATORE	315
	LETTUCE SALAD WITH CHEESE DRESSING	135
	FRUIT FOR DESSERT (OR FRUIT AND CHEESE)	100
	TOTAL:	615
7 Dinner for six	SPARKLING SANGRIA	55
	OYSTERS IMPOSTOR	60
	TERIYAKI STEAK	300
	BAKED POTATOES ROMANOFF	130
	GOLDEN DOOR COMBINATION SALAD	165
	DESSERT À TAHITI	110
	TOTAL:	820

VERY LOW CAL

GAZPACHO

(Each serving, 70 calories)

1 small cucumber, peeled and seeded
3 medium-sized tomatoes, peeled
1 teaspoon red-wine vinegar
juice of 1 lemon
1 small clove garlic,
cut up
dash of Worcestershire sauce
⅓ cup *each* diced green pepper, celery, and cucumber

Combine 1 cucumber, tomatoes, vinegar, lemon juice, garlic, and Worcestershire sauce in blender and blend until smooth. Refrigerate until ice cold. Serve topped with green pepper, celery, and cucumber.

CHILES RELLEÑOS RANCHO LA PUERTA

(Each serving, 230 calories)

1 teaspoon 100% corn-oil margarine	mildly hot kind), drained
2 eggs, separated	2 ounces (sliced about 1 × 2 × 3 inches) Monterey Jack or mild white Cheddar cheese (or ⅔ cup, shredded)
⅛ teaspoon salt	
1 tablespoon *each* unbleached flour and water, blended	
1 (4-ounce) can diced green chiles (the	chili powder

Grease with margarine a 9-inch pie pan or 2 casseroles of about 1½-cup capacity.

Beat egg whites with the salt until they hold soft peaks. Blend yolks with flour-water mixture until creamy. Gently fold whites into yolk mixture.

Spoon half the eggs into pan; distribute chiles on top, and then cheese. Cover completely with remaining egg mixture. With fingers, sprinkle enough chili powder on top to color delicately.

Bake at 325° F. for 20 to 25 minutes, or until puffy top is golden brown and feels firm. Serve at once.

TOSTADA SALAD

(Each serving, 70 calories)

½ head iceberg lettuce, cut into 4 wedges	cucumber slices, radish roses, green pepper rings, or green onions
a few garnishes typical of those used on a Mexican *tostada,* such as carrot curls, hot peppers,	Guacamole Dressing (recipe follows)
	paprika and cayenne

Arrange lettuce on 2 large plates and chill. Prepare garnishes and dressing. Pour dressing on lettuce and sprinkle with paprika and cayenne. Add garnishes at the side.

Guacamole Dressing

(Approximately 100 calories per recipe)

2 tablespoons lemon juice	sliver of garlic
1 tablespoon water	½ small, fully ripe avocado
1 teaspoon honey	salt and pepper
1 green onion	

Combine ingredients in blender and blend, adding more water, if necessary, to make a creamy thick dressing. Season to taste.

TECATE SHERBET

(Each serving, 125 calories)

1 small, fully ripe papaya or large mango, peeled and seeded, or 2 medium-sized peaches, peeled	lemon juice and orange-flavored liqueur (or orange juice with a pinch of grated peel added)
2 tablespoons *each*	2 orange slices

Cut fruit in chunks directly into blender container. Add lemon juice and liqueur. Purée, using a rubber spatula to scrape mixture down, and adding a little water if necessary.

Pour into 2 sherbet or champagne glasses and put in the freezer for 30 minutes to 1 hour. At serving time, slit each orange slice just to center and slip over glass edge.

Note: Dessert becomes too icy if frozen longer than 2 hours.

TOMATO AND CUCUMBER SALAD WITH MUSHROOMS

(Each serving, 125 calories)

1 cup ricotta cheese
1 tablespoon corn oil
   or olive oil
1 tablespoon lime or
   lemon juice
salt and pepper
2 large ripe tomatoes,
   peeled and sliced
1 crisp medium-sized
   cucumber, peeled
   and sliced
4 mushrooms, thinly
   sliced
4 red radishes, thinly
   sliced
2 green onions, thinly
   sliced

To make the dressing, combine the ricotta cheese, oil, juice, and salt and pepper in the container of a blender and blend until smooth.

Place vegetables in bowl, pour dressing over vegetables, and toss lightly.

GARDEN SPAGHETTI

(Each serving, 400 calories)

The sauce is like a stew and you eat much more of it than of the starchy accompaniment.

¼ cup chopped onion
2 cloves garlic, minced
1 tablespoon olive oil (approximate)
1½ cups unpeeled chopped eggplant
½ cup chopped cauliflower
¼ cup chopped green pepper
2 large fresh mushrooms, sliced
¼ cup minced fresh parsley
¼ teaspoon each thyme, crumbled bay leaf, and

oregano
¼ teaspoon anise or fennel seed (optional)
salt and pepper
1 (8-ounce) can tomato sauce
2 tablespoons red or white wine (approximate)
4 ounces spaghetti or noodles (green-spinach or whole-wheat variety)
2 tablespoons grated Parmesan cheese

In a large heavy pan, sauté onion and garlic in oil until limp. Add eggplant, cauliflower, green pepper, and mushrooms. Stir until vegetables begin to brown; add an additional 1 teaspoon oil if they start to stick.

Add parsley, herbs, anise, salt, pepper, and tomato sauce. Stir until mixture boils; cover and lower heat. Simmer for 30 to 40 minutes, or until eggplant and cauliflower are no longer recognizable as such but are still in chunks (not puréed). Add wine shortly before cooking is finished (more, if necessary to thin sauce).

Cook spaghetti and drain. Arrange around rim of each large plate. Heap sauce in center and sprinkle on cheese.

LEMON LIGHTNING

(Each serving, 115 calories)

- 3 tablespoons ice-cold water
- ¼ cup nonfat dry-milk powder
- 3 tablespoons cold lemon juice
- 2 teaspoons sugar
- ¼ teaspoon vanilla extract
- ⅛ teaspoon almond extract
- lemon (for grated peel)

Chill 2 sherbet dishes or custard cups. Put ice-cold water in mixing bowl and add milk. Beat with mixer until it resembles soft whipped cream. Dribble in lemon juice while beating. Sprinkle on sugar and flavoring while continuing to beat. Heap into dishes. Grate just a little peel on tops.

Eat at any stage—immediately, well-chilled, or frozen for about 1 to 1½ hours maximum (longer freezing produces ice crystals, but freezing just until firm gives rich sherbet texture).

INTERNATIONAL

SAKE MARTINI

(Each serving, 50 calories)

Many Japanese restaurants in America serve a martini made with rice wine, *sake*, which happens to be less caloric than gin or vodka.

- ¼ cup *sake*
- 1 or 2 teaspoons dry
- vermouth
- 1 strip lemon peel

Chill glasses. Shake wine with ice before pouring in. Add ice to glasses. Twist lemon to release oil into glass and drop in. Makes 1 serving.

CHICKEN LIVERS YAKITORI

(Each serving, 150 calories)

Yakitori, Japanese "shish kebab," may be made with chicken or beefsteak, as well as other ingredients such as mushrooms. Usually, *yakitori* is cooked over charcoal, but this recipe uses pan-broiling for greater ease and juiciness.

4 chicken livers, each cut into 3 pieces (if you are concerned over cholesterol, substitute parboiled skinless chicken breast)

3 green onions, white part only, cut into segments

½ green pepper, cut into 8 pieces

4 teaspoons soy sauce

2 teaspoons sugar

½ teaspoon grated fresh ginger root or ⅛ teaspoon ground ginger

1 teaspoon salad oil

salt

2 tablespoons water

Optional Japanese seasonings: *kona samsho* (ground pepper leaf) or *schichimi togarashi* (chili-sesame seasoning)

Use 4 thin metal or bamboo skewers, about 5 inches long (if they are bamboo, soak them in water so they will not burn). Thread each with one-fourth of the livers, then onion, then pepper, and so on.

In a shallow plate, blend soy sauce, sugar, ginger, and several dashes salt. Marinate skewers in sauce for about 15 minutes, turning occasionally.

Heat oil in a frying pan or, using a pastry brush, coat a griddle large enough to hold skewers. Lay skewers in pan and cook 2 to 3 minutes, brushing with marinade; turn, and cook about 3 minutes more as you brush with marinade several times, using all of marinade. Dribble in the water and turn skewers in bubbly syrup just enough to glaze. Serve hot. Sprinkle with the Japanese seasonings, if available.

MIZUTAKI FOR TWO

(Each serving, 315 calories)

Mizutaki is a Japanese dish of chicken and vegetable pieces briefly cooked in water or broth and served with dipping sauce. Usually the cooking is ceremoniously done in special pots at the table. But you'll enjoy the dish more often if you don't make such a production number of it. This recipe lets you serve up steaming bowls of *mizutaki* in just a few minutes.

Substitute ingredients of similar caloric count when necessary.

4   cups chicken broth (see page 383)
6   fresh mushrooms, sliced, or dried Oriental mushrooms *(shiitake)*
2   chicken-breast halves, skinned, boned, and cut into 12 pieces (for boning instructions, see Golden Door Breast of Chicken, page 321)
1   tablespoon soy sauce mixed with ½ teaspoon sugar
¼   cup sliced bamboo shoots
1   stalk celery, sliced diagonally into ½-inch chunks
1   carrot, sliced diagonally into ¼-inch pieces
1   (3-inch) piece Japanese white radish *(daikon)* or 1 small turnip, sliced into ¼-inch-thick rounds, each cut in half
½   green pepper, cut into 12 pieces of equal size
1   cup green vegetables (tightly packed Chinese cabbage, Chinese *bok choy,* or Swiss chard leaves cut or torn in large pieces)
4   green onions, sliced
Dipping Sauce (recipe follows)

Put broth into an 8-cup saucepan. If you use dried mushrooms, soak them in broth for about 15 minutes to soften, then cut out hard centers and cut each into 4 pieces.

Meanwhile, marinate chicken pieces in soy sauce-sugar mixture for at least 30 minutes, then drain.

Bring broth (with dried mushrooms, if used) to rolling boil; add chicken, bamboo shoots, celery, carrot, and radish. Simmer for 2 minutes. Add green pepper and fresh mushrooms, if used, and simmer for 1 more minute. Add green vegetable and green onion. Simmer about 1 more minute, or just until greens are slightly wilted.

Serve in large bowls with dipping sauce in dishes at the side. Remove foods from broth and dip in sauce. Finish by sipping broth.

Dipping Sauce

4	teaspoons toasted sesame seeds		Japanese sweet cooking wine *(mirin)*
2	tablespoons soy sauce	1	thin slice fresh ginger root or ⅛ teaspoon ground ginger
2	teaspoons lemon or lime juice		
½	small clove garlic		
1	tablespoon sherry or	1	teaspoon sugar

Pour all ingredients but 1 teaspoon sesame seeds into blender and blend. Pour into sauce dishes and sprinkle with remaining sesame seeds. (Sauce has about 100 calories.)

ORANGES IN SNOW

(Each serving, 115 calories)

In Japan a sweet similar to this, made with more sugar and agar-agar instead of gelatin, may be arranged in a black lacquer box as a gift. There the sweet is eaten at teatime. Sometimes fresh strawberry halves are used instead of mandarin oranges (or tangerines).

4	tangerines	1	tablespoon sugar
1	teaspoon unflavored gelatin	1	egg white
		⅛	teaspoon vanilla extract
1	tablespoon fresh lemon juice		
		1	drop almond extract

Squeeze 2 tangerines and add enough water to the juice to measure ⅓ cup. Combine in saucepan with gelatin, lemon juice, and sugar. Heat just to dissolve gelatin.

Beat egg white until it holds firm peaks. Still using

rotary beater, very gradually pour in lukewarm gelatin mixture, vanilla extract, and almond extract, beating until well blended. Taste and add more flavorings if you like. Pour into 2 serving dishes. Chill while doing the following:

Peel and segment the remaining 2 tangerines. Remove all membrane and cut a tiny slit in each section to press out seeds. Lay tangerines in rows on top of "snow." Chill until firm.

GOLDEN DOOR GOURMET

CITY GARDEN SALAD

(Each serving, 110 calories)

Even in a city apartment, you can grow fresh salad greens at any time of the year—in a bottle. The greens are alfalfa sprouts, which are sweeter and milder than bean sprouts, not hay-like as the name sounds. You may be able to buy sprouts, but those you grow from seed sold in health-food stores are more alive with flavor and vitamins.

Following are instructions for growing alfalfa plus a recipe for nippy dressing which enhances plain sprouts. Radishes may be a garnish. They have a complementary taste and look good chopped and mixed with your "crop."

Growing Alfalfa Sprouts: Put 1½ teaspoons seeds in a wide-mouth quart (or larger) jar. Fill with slightly warm water. The next day, place a piece of fine screen wire or a fine wire strainer very tightly over jar and drain off water.

Dampen a towel and drape around jar to almost cover the opening. This keeps light out, lets air in, and prevents seeds from drying out.

Every morning and evening for 4 to 5 days, fill jar with room-temperature water, drain, and drape with damp towel. Sprouts are ready to eat when about 1 to 1½ inches long with little green leaves.

Remove seed hulls by putting sprouts into large bowl, filling with water repeatedly as you brush floating hulls

---

off and drain sinking ones from bottom. A few hulls left in the bowl do not affect flavor, but too many are bitter. Drain sprouts. Eat right away or refrigerate in a bag with a paper towel.

Alfalfa Dressing

(185 calories per recipe)

1 tablespoon toasted sesame seeds	1½ teaspoons Dijon mustard
1 tablespoon salad oil	¼ teaspoon paprika
2 tablespoons lemon juice	1 teaspoon honey
1 tablespoon water	freshly ground black pepper

Combine all ingredients in blender and blend.

FILLET OF SOLE IN EGG BATTER

(Each serving, 100 calories)

2 (3½-ounce) pieces fillet of sole or flounder	fresh parsley
	1 tablespoon minced fresh dill
1 egg, well beaten	1 teaspoon oil
1 tablespoon minced	

Wash fish and drain. Combine egg with parsley and dill. Dip fish pieces lightly in egg on both sides (do not use all of egg). Heat oil in heavy skillet, and sauté fish until very lightly colored on bottom. Turn and sauté on other side. Remove fish to ovenproof plate covered with paper towel. Cover with aluminum foil and place in 400° F. oven for 2 to 3 minutes so that paper absorbs excess oil.

GREEN BEANS STUFATI

(Each serving, 100 calories)

½ pound fresh green beans	Golden Door seasoning salt (see page 381) and pepper
1 tablespoon 100% corn-oil margarine	

String beans and snap each into 3 pieces. Steam for 7 to 9 minutes over boiling water. Drain in colander.

In large frying pan or Chinese wok, immediately melt margarine over high heat. When it sizzles, add the beans. Stir and toss constantly about 2 minutes while adding salt and pepper. Cook just until beans are slightly more tender and very hot. Serve at once.

CARROTS CREMATE

(Each serving, 110 calories)

Borrow this low-calorie creaming technique for use with other vegetables, meats, or seafood—even a quick curry of leftovers (about 1½ cups of whatever it may be).

4 medium-sized carrots, sliced	unbleached flour
2 teaspoons salad oil	⅓ cup nonfat milk
2 teaspoons	salt and pepper
	minced parsley

Cook carrots in smallest possible amount of boiling water just until tender-crisp. Drain well and continue preparation while still hot.

Put oil in small saucepan over medium-high heat; add carrots and toss until coated and hot. Sprinkle on flour and toss to coat. Remove from heat and stir in milk. Return to low heat and cook, stirring until sauce is smooth and thick (thin with water, if necessary). Add salt and pepper to taste. Garnish with parsley and serve immediately.

Curried Variation: For a hint of curry, sprinkle in ¼ teaspoon curry powder (or more) after adding carrots to oil. (For currying leftovers, sauté several tablespoons chopped onion in the oil before adding foods. Use additional curry powder to taste.)

FRUIT AND CHEESE
FOR DESSERT

(Each serving, 50 to 100 calories)

Complementary liqueurs can be sprinkled over fresh fruit for a simple and delicious dessert. Fresh fruit alone is also satisfying. Some examples:

1	cup fresh blueberries	90	calories
1	cup fresh strawberries	50	calories
1	peach	60	calories
1	pear	100	calories
1	cup diced pineapple	80	calories
1	orange	75	calories
1	apple	80	calories
½	cantaloupe	50	calories
4-inch wedge honeydew		60	calories

One ounce of any of the following cheeses adds about 110 calories: Cheddar, Edam, Gruyère, Monterey Jack, Port Salut, Muenster.

Try different combinations of fruit and cheese. Apple is the standard with Cheddar, but you may like other cheeses even better with apples.

QUICKIE

QUICK WELSH RAREBIT

(Each serving, 330 calories)

2 teaspoons arrowroot or cornstarch
½ teaspoon *each* dry mustard, paprika, and Worcestershire sauce
1 cup (4 ounces) shredded sharp natural Cheddar cheese
¼ cup cold water
3 slices whole-wheat bread (see Tecate Bread, page 384)

Mix arrowroot and seasonings with cheese in heavy saucepan or the top of a double boiler. Stir in water.

Cook on low heat (or over boiling water), whisking or stirring constantly, until smooth and thick. (Makes ⅓ cup sauce.)

Toast bread. Cut each slice crosswise to form 4 triangles. Arrange 4 triangles around edge of each plate, spoon half the sauce inside and lay 2 triangles on sauce.

Broiled Sandwich Variation: Cool sauce until the consistency of a spread. Toast bread. Spread cheese to edges and broil until bubbly.

WALDORF SALAD

(Each serving, 175 calories)

2 small unpeeled red apples, cored and diced	onnaise (see page 380)
an equal amount of diced celery	lettuce leaves
2 tablespoons may-	2 tablespoons coarsely chopped walnuts

Toss apples and celery with the mayonnaise. Heap on lettuce-lined plates. Sprinkle walnuts on top.

BRUNCH OR LATE, LATE SUPPER

VEGETABLES BRAVADO

(Each serving, 50 to 65 calories)

cracked ice	6 cherry tomatoes
1 small celery heart or small head fresh fennel	2 sprigs parsley or watercress
1 carrot, cut in sticks or curls	Blue-Cheese Dip (recipe follows)

Fill 2 very large goblets or brandy snifters (or a bowl) with ice. Cut celery or fennel into thick slices, straight through root end, and trim tops attractively. Press upright into ice. Add carrot and tomatoes. Garnish with parsley. Serve with dip. Eat as an appetizer.

Blue·Cheese Dip

(Approximately 150 calories in recipe)

¼ cup plain, skim·milk yogurt	cheese or Roquefort
1½ teaspoons blue	½ cup pot cheese

Combine ingredients and mix well. Chill. Use ¼ cup per person.

CHICKEN CACCIATORE

(Each serving, 315 calories)

2 chicken·breast halves, skinned and boned (for boning instructions, see Golden Door Breast of Chicken, page 321)

2 teaspoons salad oil or olive oil

¼ cup chopped onion

1 small clove garlic, minced

¾ cup chopped fresh or canned tomatoes (preferably Italian plum type) plus

extra juice as needed

salt and freshly ground black pepper

¼ teaspoon each crumbled bay leaf, thyme, and marjoram

¼ cup dry white wine

½ small green pepper, cut into 12 pieces

6 fresh mushrooms (about 4 ounces), sliced

1 tablespoon 100% corn·oil margarine

Cut chicken breast into 12 pieces. In deep frying pan or pot with lid, heat 1 teaspoon oil over high heat. Sauté chicken until lightly browned and remove with a slotted spoon. Add remaining 1 teaspoon oil, onion, and garlic. Sauté until golden. Add tomatoes, salt, pepper, and herbs. Cover and simmer for 15 minutes.

Add chicken and wine; cover and simmer for 5 minutes. Add green pepper; cover and simmer for 10 minutes. Add mushrooms and margarine. Increase heat and cook rapidly, uncovered, stirring often, until mushrooms are soft and sauce looks creamy.

LETTUCE SALAD
WITH CHEESE DRESSING

(Each serving, 135 calories)

4 cups lettuce (several varieties)

3 tablespoons low-fat buttermilk

2 teaspoons corn or olive oil

1 teaspoon red- or white-wine vinegar

1 ounce blue cheese (or a mild cheese such as Monterey Jack, crumbled)

1 drop Worcestershire sauce

coarsely ground black pepper

Tear lettuce into bite-sized pieces and arrange on salad plates.

In blender, combine all remaining ingredients except pepper. Blend and pour over lettuce. Sprinkle pepper on liberally.

DINNER FOR SIX

SPARKLING SANGRIA

(Each serving, 55 calories)

For each serving
¼ cup each red wine and club soda (sparkling water)

1 tablespoon fresh orange juice
¼ thin slice each orange and lemon

Combine in tumbler or wineglass with ice cubes.
For 12 servings
Combine ⅘ quart red wine, ¾ quart club soda, ¾ cup orange juice, and 3 slices each orange and lemon, quartered.

OYSTERS IMPOSTOR

(Each serving, 60 calories)

This appetizer (which can also be a main dish) is a poor-in-calories country cousin masquerading as the much richer Oysters Rockefeller.

1	pound fresh spinach		hot-pepper sauce
12	raw oysters	1	cup shredded
	(preferably		Monterey Jack
	bluepoints), each		cheese
	scrubbed and		paprika
	opened, on a	6	lemon wedges
	half-shell		

Cook spinach slowly in its own moisture in a tightly covered pan until just slightly tender but still brilliant green. Drain, chop, and press out as much liquid as possible.

Arrange oysters in shell on baking pan. Shake 2 drops hot-pepper sauce on each. Cover each with spinach (about 1 heaping tablespoon). Sprinkle cheese on top. Sprinkle liberally with paprika.

Bake at 375° F. for about 10 minutes, or until the oysters underneath are very hot. Serve at once with lemon wedges.

TERIYAKI STEAK

(Each serving, 300 calories)

This recipe is for pan-broiling, which most chefs prefer because the meat stays juicier and a sauce is made naturally. However, the marinated meat also can be oven or charcoal broiled.

6	(4-ounce) boneless		ginger
	steaks, such as New	1	large clove garlic,
	York strip or sirloin,		crushed
	½-inch thick and	2	tablespoons dark
	trimmed of all fat		brown sugar
¼	cup soy sauce	1	tablespoon
12	paper-thin slices		polyunsaturated oil
	fresh ginger root or	2	tablespoons water
	½ teaspoon ground		

Place all ingredients except oil and water in bowl. Turn meat in marinade at least 10 minutes, or until it warms up to room temperature.

Brush the oil over a cold frying pan. Drain steaks, pat

dry with paper towel, and lay in pan. Turn heat on medium high and cook 4 minutes on each side for medium rare. Ginger slices may be browned to use as garnish.

Remove meat and keep warm on heated plates. Turn off heat. Pour the water into the pan and stir to deglaze pan. Spoon sauce, as much as you like, over steaks. Top with ginger slices.

BAKED POTATOES ROMANOFF

(Each serving, 130 calories)

6 small baking
   potatoes
½ cup each low-fat
   yogurt and low-fat
   cottage cheese

salt and pepper
1 (1-ounce) jar black
   caviar (lumpfish
   type is fine)

Bake potatoes at 375° F. until tender. Meanwhile, mix yogurt and cheese in blender until thickened like sour cream.

Slit each potato down the middle lengthwise and twice crosswise. Press from both sides to puff potato upward and spread open. Season with salt and pepper. Spoon on yogurt-cheese. Top each potato with a dab of caviar.

GOLDEN DOOR
COMBINATION SALAD

(Each serving, 165 calories)

3 cups torn lettuce,
   preferably a mixture
   of several kinds
½ cup each raw cauli-
   flowerettes, broccoli
   flowerettes, raw
   bean sprouts, and
   slivered green or
   red pepper
6 tablespoons corn or

olive oil
¼ cup fresh lemon
   juice
1 teaspoon Dijon
   mustard
1 clove garlic, crushed
salt and pepper
2 fully ripe tomatoes,
   chopped

Put lettuce and vegetables in large mixing bowl. Blend all remaining ingredients *except* tomato for dressing. Serve in individual salad bowls. Top each with a spoonful of tomato.

DESSERT À TAHITI

(Each serving, 110 calories)

2 cups chopped fresh pineapple	1 teaspoon vanilla extract
3 eggs	1½ teaspoons orange- flavored liqueur
1 cup nonfat milk	
2 tablespoons sugar	orange (for grated peel)

In the top of a double boiler, combine eggs, milk, and sugar; whisk to blend egg thoroughly. Cook over boiling water. When mixture begins to thicken, stir continuously until the consistency of heavy cream—the custard will not get very thick. Remove from heat and blend in liqueur and vanilla extract. Cool to room temperature.

Pour custard over pineapple. Grate a little orange peel for a garnish. Chill before serving (either in the pineapple shell or in 2 champagne or sherbet glasses).

WEEK III
OF DINNER MENUS
FOR WEIGHT REDUCTION

		CALORIES
1	SPINACH SOUP	170
Very low cal	MEAT-PATTY PLATTER	335
	ZIGZAG MELON ESCONDIDO	40
	TOTAL:	545
2	COLD CUCUMBER SOUP	90
Vegetarian	MARINATED VEGETABLE MAZA	70
	TABBOULEH SALAD	280
	CHEESE WEDGE	110
	TOTAL:	550

		CALORIES
3 International	OYSTERS AT SEA	45
	LILY POND WAN	35
	FISH SHIOYAKI	300
	CUCUMBER-CELERY SUNOMO	40
	FRUIT FOR DESSERT	100
	TOTAL:	520

4 Golden Door Gourmet	MEDITERRANEAN TOMATO SALAD	65
	CHICKEN PAPRIKASH	270
	EGGPLANT HUNGARIAN	105
	SLIM PEACH MELBA	85
	TOTAL:	525

5 Quickie	GUACAMOLE-STUFFED MUSHROOMS	110
	POT-AU-FEU	430
	TIPSY PINEAPPLE HAWAIIAN	115
	TOTAL:	655

6 Brunch or late, late supper	FRESH GREEN BEAN SALAD	130
	SHRIMP-STUFFED FISH	265
	COEUR À LA CRÈME	175
	TOTAL:	570

7 Dinner for six	FRUIT-FROSTED WINE	55
	CAVIAR MOUSSE	75
	FOIL-BAKED CHICKEN	175
	BAKED STUFFED TOMATO	200
	RAW MUSHROOM SALAD	145
	BANANA ICE CREAM	100
	TOTAL:	750

SPINACH SOUP

(Each serving, 170 calories)

1 pound fresh spinach	whole-wheat flour
1 tablespoon 100% corn-oil margarine	2 cups chicken broth (see recipe page 383)
¼ cup finely chopped onion	salt and pepper
1 clove garlic, minced	2 tablespoons grated Parmesan cheese
1 teaspoon	

Wash spinach carefully to remove any grit or sand, and chop.

In a heavy skillet, melt the margarine and sauté the onion and garlic until golden. Add the spinach. Cover tightly and steam over low heat for about 3 minutes, or until spinach is wilted. Stir in the flour and add chicken broth. Simmer for 5 minutes. Season to taste with salt and pepper.

Purée the soup in a blender; reheat to serve, and sprinkle with Parmesan cheese.

MEAT-PATTY PLATTER

(Each serving, 335 calories)

½ pound ground round steak (without fat)	2 thin slices Monterey Jack or Swiss cheese
2 lettuce leaves	catsup and/or mayonnaise (see pages 377 and 380)
1 large tomato cut into 4 slices	
watercress sprigs	

Form beef into 2 oblong patties. Pat firmly with the flat side of a wide knife blade and then score gently in a crisscross pattern on both sides while rounding edges a bit. (This makes meat look attractive and also keeps it from cracking as it cooks.)

For each serving, arrange on a dinner plate a lettuce

leaf topped with 2 tomato slices and a bed of water-cress.

Cook patties in a heated frying pan for 2 minutes; turn and cover. Cook until hot, uncover, and lay cheese on top. Cover again and cook about 2 minutes more, until patty has browned on bottom and cheese melts a little. Lay meat beside watercress and decorate with a dollop of catsup and/or mayonnaise.

ZIGZAG MELON ESCONDIDO

(Each serving, 40 calories)

2 lengthwise wedges cantaloupe, honeydew, or Persian melon	2 sprigs fresh mint (optional)
	2 large strawberries
	2 lemon wedges

Zigzag each wedge: First, at each tip make crosswise cut just to the rind. Then slice inward from the cut close to rind all the way underneath to reach the other end, and free melon in one piece.

Put melon, still on rind, on a plate. Cut crosswise into 6 pieces of equal width. Pull the first about ½ inch to one side, the next ½ inch to the other side, and so on to zigzag all pieces. Lay mint, berry, and lemon in a row at the center of each melon.

Pineapple Variation: Fresh pineapple can also be prepared this way.

VEGETARIAN

COLD CUCUMBER SOUP

(Each serving, 90 calories)

This quick blender combination makes a soup you can sip like a cocktail before dinner.

1 cup low-fat yogurt	⅛ teaspoon dried dill weed or several sprigs fresh dill
½ cup water	
½ small clove garlic	
8 fresh mint leaves or	1 cucumber
¼ teaspoon dried crumbled mint	salt

Put yogurt, water, garlic, and herbs in blender. Cut a small slice of unpeeled cucumber off either end and reserve for garnish. Peel rest of cucumber, cut in half, scoop out and discard seeds. Cut in small pieces into blender container. Blend until creamy. Add salt to taste.

Serve in cocktail or champagne glasses. Cut a slit to the center of each reserved cucumber slice and slip over glass rim. Chill thoroughly. Serve with a floating ice cube.

MARINATED VEGETABLE MAZA

(Each serving, 70 calories)

Throughout the Near and Middle East, *maza* or *meze* means appetizer.

2 raw turnips, thinly sliced

2 carrots, scraped and thinly sliced

½ cup pickled-beet juice or the following blend: ½ cup juice drained from cooked beets, mixed with 1 tablespoon vinegar, 1 teaspoon sugar, and a sprinkling of salt

Marinate vegetables in beet juice for at least 15 minutes or for several hours, turning to make sure turnips become deep pink and carrots deep red-orange. Drain before serving.

TABBOULEH SALAD

(Each serving, 280 calories)

This Arabic salad has universal appeal. With a little effort you can find bulgur almost anywhere now. Bulgur comes in three forms—large almost-whole grains (the type also to use for pilaf), medium-sized cracked, and very finely cracked. The medium size is the best for *tabbouleh,* but the more frequently found large size works fine.

½ cup bulgur

2 large, fully ripe tomatoes, finely chopped

1 small green bell pepper, finely chopped

1 small cucumber, peeled and finely chopped

6 small green onions, including part of tops, finely chopped

6 radishes, finely chopped

1 cup finely minced parsley (about 2 large bunches)

1 tablespoon minced fresh mint leaves

Dressing (recipe follows)

lemon wedges for garnish, and lettuce leaves

nutmeg (optional)

Optional garnishes: tomato wedges, green-pepper rings, cucumber slices, small green onions, radish roses, parsley, or mint leaves

Cover bulgur with water by at least 1 inch and soak until soft but still slightly crunchy—about 30 minutes. Strain and press out excess water.

Combine with chopped vegetables, parsley, and mint. Dribble dressing over and toss with fork. Let salad marinate for about 15 minutes, or chill as long as several hours. Make beds of lettuce leaves on large plates, heap salad in centers, add lemon wedges and optional garnishes. Pass nutmeg to sprinkle on salad, if desired.

Dressing

2 tablespoons olive oil

2 tablespoons fresh lemon juice

½ teaspoon salt

½ teaspoon allspice (optional)

½ teaspoon dry mustard

¼ teaspoon freshly ground black pepper

Dash of hot-pepper sauce or cayenne

1 small clove garlic, pressed

Combine ingredients and mix well. Pour over salad.

OYSTERS AT SEA

(Each serving, 45 calories)

For serving you will need 2 plates or bowls, preferably pottery or straw; pebbles, similar to those sold for flower arrangements; and 2 tiny sauce cups or extra oyster shells.

6 raw oysters, on the half-shell	½ teaspoon soy sauce
1 tablespoon each Japanese rice-wine vinegar (or regular distilled white vinegar) and fresh lemon juice	1 teaspoon grated Japanese white radish *(daikon)* or regular red radish or turnip
	¼ teaspoon grated fresh ginger root

Line plates with pebbles. On each plate arrange 3 oysters on half-shells, with a sauce cup. Blend vinegar and lemon juice, and sprinkle oysters with one-fourth of mixture. For dipping sauce, blend the remaining vinegar-lemon mixture with soy sauce, radish, and ginger. Pour into sauce dishes.

LILY POND WAN

(Each serving, 35 calories)

Wan is very clear soup containing tidbits of colorful vegetables that create a still life when presented in a simple classic soup bowl of black or Chinese-red lacquer.

2 cups clear chicken broth (see recipe page 383) or Japanese *dashi* broth (instructions follow)	carrot
	2 very small spinach leaves or watercress sprigs
2 paper-thin slices	1 paper-thin slice lemon, cut in half

Heat broth, add carrot, and simmer for 1 minute, or just until carrot turns bright orange. Pour broth into Japanese bowls and put a carrot slice in each. Slip leaf and lemon into each "pond." Serve hot. Sip from the bowl.

Instructions for Dashi Broth: Buy a box of ingredients labeled *dashi-no-moto* soup stock (it comes in either pellet form or in little bags resembling tea bags). Many supermarkets carry this in the gourmet or Oriental section. Brew according to package directions. For clear broth, do not press bag; remove gently. Let broth cool and settle. Pour off clear top for Lily Pond Wan. Refrigerate or freeze remainder. *Dashi* is the broth you should use for sukiyaki or tempura dipping sauce.

FISH SHIOYAKI

(Each serving, 300 calories)

The Japanese method of *shio* (salt) *yaki* (broiling) produces the most delicious fish. For genuine *shioyaki* the fish must have skin on it. Salt is sprinkled on skin only, never on the flesh. That is why the large amount of salt does not make the fish taste salty.

2 small whole fish (about 1/3 pound each) or 1 larger fish weighing 2/3 pound	(lettuce for delicate fish, cabbage for stronger-flavored types)
salt	1 thick slice each orange and lemon, both cut in half
2/3 cup finely shredded lettuce or cabbage	

Fresh- or saltwater fish may be used. A good choice is rainbow trout or a sea fish of similar size and shape. Small whole fish with head and tail intact cook more easily and look best. But fish without head or tail, or pieces with skin on can be used. Fish must be fully cleaned internally, and scaled.

Fish should be at room temperature and patted dry with paper towel before cooking. Oil head and tail to prevent drying.

To cook, line broiler pan with foil. Preheat broiler with rack about 6 inches below. (Fish could also be charcoal-broiled.)

Cut about 3 diagonal slashes at intervals on each side

of fish, just through skin. Lay fish on pan and sprinkle *heavily* with salt. (If you like to eat fish skin, use about twice as much salt as you would use for meat. If you don't eat the skin, salt even more heavily.) *Do not* salt inside fish or on flesh anywhere.

Broil about 3 to 4 minutes for ⅓-pound fish or 5 minutes for ⅔-pound fish. Turn, again salt heavily, cover tail with foil to prevent burning; broil about the same amount of time again. Skin of fish will be blistered and crispy; salt will be partially white and somewhat browned.

Meanwhile, prepare serving plates with a row of shredded vegetable down one side of each. Lay fish beside vegetable; place orange half between, and lemon half atop orange. Serve both fish and salad completely plain, or with a few drops of citrus juice from the garnish.

CUCUMBER-CELERY SUNOMO

(Each serving, 40 calories)

Sunomo is the Japanese word for dishes resembling salads.

1 cucumber	2 teaspoons *sake* (Japanese rice wine) or dry sherry (optional)
2 stalks celery	
3 tablespoons Japanese rice-wine vinegar or regular distilled white vinegar	
	¼ teaspoon salt
	¼ teaspoon grated fresh ginger root (optional)
1 tablespoon water	
2 teaspoons sugar	

Prepare the garnishes first: Cut 2 "ribbons" of cucumber peel about 6 inches long and ½ inch wide. Trim edges evenly. Tie each in a single, loose knot. Also reserve 2 tiny celery-leaf clusters.

Finish peeling cucumber; cut in half lengthwise; scoop out seeds and discard them. Slice paper-thin. Slice celery diagonally paper-thin. Toss together in bowl.

Blend remaining ingredients and pour over salad. Toss, taste, and add salt, if necessary. Chill.

Heap into two small bowls. Perch cucumber knot on each mound and tuck celery leaves inside knot.

GOLDEN DOOR GOURMET

MEDITERRANEAN TOMATO SALAD

(Each serving, 65 calories)

2 large romaine leaves
1 large, fully ripe tomato, cut into 4 slices
salt and pepper

fresh parsley
2 lemon wedges
1 teaspoon fresh or ¼ teaspoon dried oregano
2 teaspoons olive oil

For each serving: Lay leaf on plate, top with 2 tomato slices, and season with salt and pepper. Tuck parsley sprig at side and garnish with 1 lemon wedge.

Mince ½ teaspoon parsley and mix with oregano. Sprinkle on tomatoes, then dribble oil on. Squeeze lemon on for tartness as desired.

CHICKEN PAPRIKASH

(Each serving, 270 calories)

Paprika is the most typical Hungarian seasoning. Hungarian cooks use it to flavor and thicken sauces, as well as for color. Ground from dried capsicum peppers, paprika comes in a wide spectrum of pungency, from very hot to sweetly mild.

1 pound frying-chicken pieces (white meat)
½ cup water
¼ pound fresh mushrooms, sliced
½ onion, sliced
½ cup chopped green

pepper
1 sliver garlic, minced
pinch of pepper
½ cup plain low-fat yogurt
1 tablespoon sweet Hungarian paprika

Place chicken pieces, skin side down, in a skillet. Add 2 tablespoons water. Cover and cook very slowly over medium heat until the water evaporates and the chicken begins to brown in its own fat. Add mushrooms, onion, green pepper, and garlic and brown slowly. Pour off fat that has accumulated in the pan.

Add the remaining water. Cover and simmer for 35 to 40 minutes or until chicken is tender. Remove chicken from pan and keep warm.

Skim any fat from the surface of the pan juices. Stir in yogurt and paprika and cook over low heat until warmed through. *Do not boil.*

Pour sauce over chicken and serve immediately.

EGGPLANT HUNGARIAN

(Each serving, 105 calories)

1 small eggplant (preferably long Italian style) Golden Door seasoning salt (see page 381)	oregano 2 teaspoons polyunsaturated oil

Wash the eggplant, remove the ends, and slice lengthwise. Make shallow crosswise incisions with a knife. Sprinkle with seasonings and a teaspoon of polyunsaturated oil. Bake in a 350° F. oven for 30 to 40 minutes. Serve immediately.

SLIM PEACH MELBA

(Each serving, 85 calories)

2 fresh peaches, peeled and halved ¼ cup low-fat yogurt 2 teaspoons honey several dashes of	nutmeg ¼ cup chopped fresh strawberries or raspberries lime (for grated peel)

Arrange 1 peach half in each of 2 sherbet or champagne glasses.

Into blender put yogurt, 1 teaspoon honey, nutmeg,

and 1 peach half, cut in small pieces. Purée. Chop last peach half and add to sauce (do not blend). Pour into glasses.

Blend berries with remaining 1 teaspoon honey and spoon into peach centers. Grate on lime peel.

QUICKIE

GUACAMOLE-STUFFED MUSHROOMS

(Each serving, 110 calories)

¼ pound medium-sized mushrooms
1½ teaspoons lemon juice
½ teaspoon salt
½ ripe avocado

1 teaspoon finely minced onion
dash of hot-pepper sauce
1 tablespoon diced tomato

Wipe mushrooms clean. Remove stems and reserve for other uses. Brush insides of caps with half the lemon juice and sprinkle with a bit of salt. Mash avocado and blend in remaining lemon juice, salt, onion, and hot-pepper sauce. Mix well. Fill each cap with a tablespoon of the mixture and garnish with some diced tomato.

POT-AU-FEU

(Each serving, 430 calories)

This dish must be prepared the day before it is to be served. After it is refrigerated overnight, the fat, which has risen to the top, is easy to remove. The dish improves in flavor by sitting for 12 to 24 hours.

For two servings, only ½ the meat is served. The remaining meat is excellent in a cold salad. Any leftover broth can be frozen and used as a soup base.

1 pound beef rump or round (lean only), cut into cubes	bag or placed in a tea ball)
1 teaspoon salt	1½ cups mixed coarsely chopped vegetables (onion, carrots, celery, white turnips, parsnips— whatever suits your taste)
1 *bouquet garni* (1 bay leaf, ¼ teaspoon thyme, ½ teaspoon peppercorns, 1 clove garlic, 3 whole cloves, 4 sprigs parsley, and a few celery leaves tied in a cheesecloth	2 leeks, white part only, sliced
	2 carrots, peeled and quartered
	2 potatoes, washed

Place the meat in a heavy soup kettle with water to cover. Add the salt and *bouquet garni*. Bring to a boil, skimming the foam from the top as it rises. Reduce the heat and simmer, covered, until the meat is almost tender, about 3 hours. Discard the *bouquet garni* and correct the seasoning. Refrigerate.

When ready to serve, remove the accumulated fat from the top and reheat. Add the vegetables, except the potatoes, and simmer until tender, about 30 minutes. Meanwhile cook the potatoes separately, until tender. Peel, quarter, and add to pot-au-feu. Serve half of the meat.

Some people prefer their pot-au-feu served with the meat in the broth, but the French prefer to sip the broth first and then eat the meat. Serve with *cornichons* (small European sour pickles) and Dijon mustard or horseradish sauce.

TIPSY PINEAPPLE HAWAIIAN

(Each serving, 115 calories)

½ small fresh pineapple	liqueur (optional)
2 teaspoons rum or orange-flavored	2 tablespoons shredded coconut, plain or toasted

Cut pineapple in half lengthwise right through leaves and reserve half for other uses. Cut other half in two lengthwise, again right through leaves. With a small knife, cut out cores. Cut between rind and fruit to loosen completely, but leave in place. Cut fruit in chunks by slicing each serving lengthwise through the middle and crosswise five or six times.

Sprinkle liqueur along centers. Top with coconut.

BRUNCH OR LATE, LATE SUPPER

FRESH GREEN BEAN SALAD

(Each serving, 130 calories)

¾ pound green beans (young, tender, and fresh)

1 teaspoon finely chopped shallots

1 teaspoon chopped fresh parsley

1 to 2 tablespoons vinaigrette dressing (see Golden Door Combination Salad, page 341)

lettuce
pimiento strips

Cut the ends from the beans; remove strings and slice beans lengthwise. Blanch in boiling salted water for 2 to 3 minutes. Drain and cool immediately (the beans must still be green and crisp). Add the shallots and parsley. When ready to serve, blend in the dressing. Serve the salad on a bed of lettuce with additional parsley sprinkled on top. Decorate each portion with crossed strips of red pimiento.

SHRIMP-STUFFED FISH

(Each serving, 265 calories)

2 (⅓-pound) fish fillets, such as flounder or sole

½ cup (about 2 ounces) tiny shrimp or larger shrimp, cut up

2 fresh mushrooms, halved and sliced

5 saltines, crushed

3 tablespoons nonfat dry-milk powder

1 egg

2 teaspoons lemon juice

salt and pepper

2 teaspoons polyunsaturated oil

1 tablespoon minced parsley

1 tablespoon dry white wine or dry vermouth

Lay each fillet flat. With small sharp-pointed knife, cut a slit lengthwise down the center, about halfway through only. Make pockets for stuffing on both sides of slit by cutting from within slit nearly through to each edge. (The fillet, slit with pockets on each side, should resemble wrapping used for individual packets of facial tissue.)

Combine shrimp, mushrooms, crackers, milk powder, egg, lemon juice, and salt and pepper to taste. Blend with a fork.

Oil 2 individual oblong ramekins or 2 pieces of aluminum foil. Lay fish in (bring foil up around sides to make a sort of boat) and lay on baking pan. Stuff fish with shrimp mixture. Tuck ends of fish under; brush sides with 2 teaspoons oil, sprinkle parsley over stuffing, and pour wine into container.

Bake uncovered at 375° F. for 10 to 15 minutes, or until fish flakes easily when tested with fork.

COEUR À LA CRÈME

(Each serving, 175 calories)

This is a low-calorie version of the classic French dessert.

½ cup low-fat creamed cottage cheese	pinch of salt
	2 tablespoons sugar
½ (3-ounce) package Neufchatel cheese, slightly softened	¾ cup fresh strawberries

In the morning, thoroughly blend cheeses, salt, and sugar in a bowl. Refrigerate.

About 15 minutes before serving, form the cheese into a heart shape, place on a platter, and surround with berries.

DINNER FOR SIX

FRUIT-FROSTED WINE

(Each serving, 55 calories)

⅘ quart dry white wine, like Chablis, chilled	chilled
	1 large peach, cut in 12 slices
1 quart club soda,	12 large strawberries

Just before serving, combine ingredients in large glass pitcher. Serve over ice. Makes 12 servings (two glasses per person).

CAVIAR MOUSSE

(Each ¼ cup, 55 calories; 20 calories per 2 crackers)

1 envelope (1 tablespoon) un-flavored gelatin
2 tablespoons cold water
½ cup boiling water
1 tablespoon lemon juice
2 tablespoons mayonnaise (see page 380)

dash of hot-pepper sauce
2 teaspoons minced shallots
4 ounces (½ cup) red caviar or chopped olives
2 cups plain low-fat yogurt
watercress
melba toast or rye thins

Soften gelatin in cold water. Add boiling water and stir until dissolved. Cool slightly, then stir in lemon juice, mayonnaise, hot-pepper sauce, shallots, caviar, and yogurt. Rinse 3½- to 4-cup mold with cold water; drain, and spoon in caviar mixture. Chill until set (2 to 3 hours). Unmold and serve on a bed of watercress, accompanied by crackers.

FOIL-BAKED CHICKEN

(Each serving, 175 calories)

6 small whole chicken breasts or 6 large halves, skinned and boned
salt
6 tablespoons minced celery
6 tablespoons minced

onion
2 tablespoons minced fresh parsley
6 tablespoons lemon juice
6 tablespoons dry white wine or dry vermouth

Cut six squares (18 × 18 inches) of aluminum foil. Place a breast on each square and sprinkle with salt, celery, onion, and parsley. Add lemon juice and wine to each package. Pull four corners of foil up to make a tight bundle around chicken. Place packages in shallow baking pan and bake at 375° F. for 35 minutes. Serve hot, or chilled with juice jelled around chicken.

BAKED STUFFED TOMATO

(Each serving, 200 calories)

6 large tomatoes	¾ teaspoon tarragon
1½ cups diced Monterey Jack cheese	¾ teaspoon sweet basil
	pepper and salt
¾ cup dry bread crumbs	3 cloves garlic, pressed

Cut tops off tomatoes and scoop out centers. Seed and chop the pulp. Lightly sprinkle the inside of each scooped-out tomato with salt. Mix tomato pulp with remaining ingredients, and spoon into the tomatoes. Bake at 375° F. for 15 minutes, or until bubbly.

RAW MUSHROOM SALAD

(Each serving, 145 calories)

36 fresh mushrooms, thinly sliced	2 tablespoons minced chives
2 tablespoons lemon juice	2 tablespoons minced fresh parsley
2 tablespoons wine vinegar	Golden Door seasoning salt (see page 381)
4 tablespoons polyunsaturated oil	freshly ground black pepper
2 tablespoons chopped green onion	lettuce leaves
	alfalfa sprouts (see page 385)

Place mushrooms in a bowl. Toss with lemon juice and vinegar. Add oil, green onion, chives, parsley, seasoning salt, and pepper. Toss again. Chill before serving.

When ready to serve, select a few handsome leaves of lettuce and place on two individual salad plates. Cover with a small mound of alfalfa sprouts and the marinated mushrooms.

BANANA ICE CREAM

(Each serving, 100 calories)

6 small bananas (fully ripe but not overripe)
lemon juice
1½ teaspoons vanilla extract
¾ cup cold nonfat milk or water (approximate)

Peel bananas; cut out any brown spots and cut off tips. Carefully remove all tiny strings down the sides or any imperfection (black spot or bruise). Squeeze lemon juice all over to prevent discoloration. Wrap each banana tightly in plastic wrap. Freeze solid. Chill 2 sherbet or champagne glasses.

At serving time, put vanilla and milk into the blender container. Quickly cut bananas into small chunks directly into container. Blend; turn blender on and off and scrape mixture down with a rubber spatula, as necessary, until smooth and creamy. Add more cold milk if ice cream gets too thick to blend fully. Pour into chilled glasses. (Dessert may be held in freezer a few minutes before serving, but do not refreeze—ice crystals form.)

Banana-Strawberry Variation: Combine 1 frozen banana with about 6 large frozen strawberries.

WEEK IV
OF DINNER MENUS
FOR WEIGHT REDUCTION

		CALORIES
1 Very low cal	BROILED SHRIMP	210
	GREEN SALAD WITH	
	ONION AND ORANGE	90
	PALACE MUHALLEBI	130
	TOTAL:	430
2 Vegetarian	WATER CHESTNUTS	
	RUMAKI	75
	FRESH FRUIT PLATE	
	WITH PEACH DRESSING	275
	BISCUIT TORTONI	115
	TOTAL:	465
3 International	GREEK AVGOLEMONO	
	SOUP	75
	CRUSTY LAMB CHOPS	400
	SPINACH SALAD WITH	
	SUNFLOWER DRESSING	95
	BROILED PAPAYA	110
	TOTAL:	680
4 Golden Door Gourmet	MUSHROOM-STUFFED	
	MUSHROOMS	80
	SOLE ALL'AGRO DI LIMONE	260
	ASPARAGUS MIMOSA	80
	STRAWBERRIES MYSTERY	95
	TOTAL:	515
5 Quickie	VIRGIN MARY COCKTAIL	
	WITH CELERY	25
	CELERY ROOT AND	
	APPLE SALAD	100
	FAST FONDUE WITH	
	SKINNY DIPPERS	430
	PRUNE COMPOTE IN PORT	185
	TOTAL:	740

		CALORIES
6	RADISHES ON ICE	55
Brunch or late,	CHIC CONSOMMÉ	45
late supper	SVELTE CHICKEN	205
	PEAS AU NATUREL	65
	CELESTIAL STRAWBERRY	
	ANGEL CAKE	175
	TOTAL:	545

7	WHITE-WINE SPRITZER	
Dinner for six	*(see page 320)*	45
	SMOKED SALMON SPEARS	55
	BROILED CHICKEN WITH	
	MUSTARD SAUCE	270
	GLAZED NEW POTATOES	90
	MEDITERRANEAN	
	TOMATO SALAD	65
	SIMPLY CHEESECAKE	175
	TOTAL:	700

VERY LOW CAL

BROILED SHRIMP

(Each serving, 210 calories)

6 very large (about 5
inches long) raw,
unpeeled shrimp or
about ⅔ pound
largest size

2 tablespoons 100%

corn-oil margarine

1 tablespoon lemon
juice

1 tablespoon white
wine, dry vermouth,
or water

Prepare shrimp to be broiled in shells with tails intact this way: Slit each shrimp lengthwise through shell down vein just far enough to butterfly (lay flat open); clean vein. Loosen meat within shell and score it lightly with knife blade in crisscross pattern to prevent curling. Lay each, shell side down, on foil-lined broiler pan. Preheat broiler.

Melt margarine in small saucepan. Brush about half on shrimp. Add lemon juice and wine to remaining margarine and heat (don't simmer).

Broil shrimp 6 inches from heat for about 5 minutes, or until very pink and beginning to brown (brush once with margarine-lemon mixture). Pour remaining hot mixture into small cups and serve as dipping sauce.

GREEN SALAD
WITH ONION AND ORANGE

(Each serving, 90 calories)

1 clove garlic, halved	1 small orange, peeled and thinly sliced
3 cups watercress sprigs or small pieces of curly endive or romaine (approximate)	1 tablespoon corn oil or olive oil
2 thin slices sweet white or red onion, separated into rings, or 2 green onions, thinly sliced	1 teaspoon each red-wine vinegar and red wine (or water)
	pinch of dry mustard
	salt and pepper

Rub salad bowl with garlic. Add greens, onion, and orange. Blend remaining ingredients. Dribble over greens as you toss with fork. Add more vinegar, if needed.

PALACE MUHALLEBI

(Each serving, 130 calories)

The simple milk pudding Muhallebi is as popular in Turkey as fruit gelatin is in the United States.

4 teaspoons cornstarch	pods, each slit on one side
2 tablespoons sugar	several dashes of salt
¼ cup water	1 tablespoon finely chopped toasted blanched almonds
1 cup cold nonfat milk	
5 whole cardamom	

In heavy saucepan mix cornstarch with sugar and stir in water; add milk, cardamom, and salt. Cook over very low heat for about 10 minutes, stirring often (do not simmer). When pudding begins to thicken, stir constantly until thick. Remove from heat and discard cardamom.

Pour into sherbet or parfait glasses and cover with wax paper to prevent skin from forming. Serve warm, chilled, or the Turkish way—at room temperature with almonds on top.

VEGETARIAN

WATER CHESTNUTS RUMAKI

(Each serving, 75 calories)

| 16 | whole canned water chestnuts, well drained | ¼ | teaspoon grated fresh ginger root, or several dashes ground ginger |
| 1 | tablespoon soy sauce | 2 | teaspoons sugar |

Marinate chestnuts in soy sauce and ginger for at least 10 minutes. Drain well in strainer. Preheat oven to 450° F. or preheat broiler.

Put chestnuts on plate and sprinkle with sugar, rolling each chestnut to coat thoroughly. Spear each with a pick (for broiling, spear at sides so picks do not stick upward and burn).

Bake on a foil-lined pan for about 5 minutes, or until hot and glazed. Or broil 4 inches from heat for about 2 minutes, turn, and broil a minute or so more until glazed.

FRESH FRUIT PLATE
WITH PEACH DRESSING

(Each serving, 275 calories)

1 small head butter lettuce, or other soft lettuce

2 large fresh peaches, peeled, halved, and pitted

1 cup low-fat yogurt

½ cup low-fat cottage cheese

1 medium-sized grapefruit, peeled and divided into 6 wedges

½ medium-sized cantaloupe, peeled and cut into 6 wedges

10 large strawberries

1 bunch watercress

ground nutmeg

2 mint sprigs (optional)

For each serving, make a bed of the outside lettuce leaves on a dinner plate. Coarsely shred remaining lettuce. Place a small custard cup or Oriental teacup in center of plate. Heap shredded lettuce into and over it. Place 1 peach half, pitted side up, on top of each cup.

For dressing, combine yogurt and remaining 2 peach halves in blender and purée. Chill.

Form cottage cheese into 2 balls. Place on each peach half. Around side of each plate, arrange 3 grapefruit wedges, 3 cantaloupe wedges, and 5 strawberries. Fill spaces between fruit groups with watercress.

Pour dressing over peach mound. Sprinkle liberally with nutmeg and add a mint sprig on top.

BISCUIT TORTONI

(Each serving, 115 calories)

¼ cup each nonfat dry-milk powder and ice-cold water

2 teaspoons fresh lemon juice

5 teaspoons sugar

1 teaspoon sherry

¼ teaspoon vanilla extract

⅛ teaspoon almond extract

1 tablespoon slivered blanched almonds, toasted

Combine milk powder and water in mixing bowl. Beat with an electric mixer until mixture resembles softly whipped cream. Continue to beat while sprinkling in lemon juice, sugar, sherry, vanilla extract, and almond extract. Beat until smooth and creamy like a light meringue. Heap into chilled custard cups or large paper baking cups in a chilled muffin pan. Put in freezer while preparing nuts.

Whirl almonds in blender to grind (or chop as finely as possible). Sprinkle over desserts to cover tops completely. Tortoni may be eaten partially frozen, or fully frozen (it takes about 1 hour). However, freezing more than about 1½ hours may produce ice crystals which spoil the smooth texture.

INTERNATIONAL
GREEK AVGOLEMONO SOUP
(Each serving, 75 calories)

1	egg	grated lemon peel,
1½	tablespoons fresh lemon juice	minced parsley, or fresh mint for
2	cups chicken broth (see page 383)	garnish

In a bowl, blend egg and lemon juice. Heat broth until boiling, then remove from heat. Beat a small amount of the hot broth into the eggs, then add to remaining broth, beating constantly. Heat through, continuing to stir constantly. Serve hot. Sprinkle one or more of the garnishes on top.

CRUSTY LAMB CHOPS
(Each serving of two chops, 400 calories)

2	tablespoons nonfat milk	polyunsaturated oil
1	tablespoon whole-wheat flour	4 loin lamb chops (5 ounces each before
2	tablespoons plain toasted wheat germ	trimming), trimmed of all fat, at room
2	teaspoons	temperature
		salt and pepper

Put milk in bowl. On a plate, blend flour and wheat germ. Pour 1 teaspoon oil in small frying pan over medium heat and turn pan to distribute evenly.

Dip each chop in milk, then coat in flour-wheat germ mixture, which has been seasoned with salt and pepper. Broil about 5 minutes, or until brown and crusty. Turn, adding the remaining 1 teaspoon oil. Broil about 5 minutes more, or until done to your liking.

SPINACH SALAD
WITH SUNFLOWER DRESSING

(Each serving, 95 calories)

4 cups torn fresh spinach leaves (or whole small inside leaves, for a more elegant salad)
2 tablespoons olive oil

1 tablespoon lemon juice
tarragon and nutmeg
lemon (for grated peel)
2 tablespoons sunflower seeds

Put greens in bowl. Mix oil, lemon juice, several pinches of pulverized tarragon, and a dash of nutmeg. Grate a tiny bit of lemon peel onto greens. Dribble on dressing and toss with fork. Divide into two salad bowls. Sprinkle sunflower seeds on top.

BROILED PAPAYA

(Each serving, 110 calories)

1 ripe but firm papaya (about 8 ounces)
1 tablespoon lemon or lime juice
2 teaspoons dark

brown sugar
2 tablespoons shredded coconut
lemon or lime wedges

Cut papaya in half lengthwise and discard seeds. Cut 8 slashes around sides (into fruit, but not through to the skin). Sprinkle juice over tops and into cavities. Sprinkle with sugar.

Preheat broiler. Broil fruit 6 inches from heat for about 5 minutes, or until very hot. Sprinkle coconut into cavities and broil again for about 1 or 2 minutes, or just until coconut is toasted. Watch carefully—coconut can burn quickly. Serve hot with lemon wedges.

MUSHROOM-STUFFED MUSHROOMS

(Each serving, 80 calories)

6 large mushrooms (at least 2 inches wide)
1 thin slice onion, chopped
2 teaspoons 100% corn-oil margarine
2 tablespoons dry vermouth or water
salt and pepper
¼ teaspoon each basil and oregano

Remove mushroom stems and chop. In a saucepan sauté stems and onion in margarine until they begin to brown. Spoon into mushroom caps and return to pan. Pour in vermouth. Sprinkle seasonings on caps.

Cover and simmer for about 10 minutes, or until about 1 tablespoon liquid remains. Serve hot with liquid spooned over.

SOLE ALL'AGRO DI LIMONE

(Each serving, 260 calories)

⅔ pound fillet of sole or other mild white fish (preferably 2 pieces of equal size)
salt and pepper
1 tablespoon unbleached flour
2 teaspoons corn or olive oil
1 tablespoon 100%
corn-oil margarine
1½ teaspoons lemon juice
¼ cup dry white wine or dry vermouth
1 tablespoon minced parsley
4 thin lemon slices
paprika

Sprinkle the fish with salt and pepper and lightly coat with flour. In a small frying pan, heat the oil over medium-high heat. Sprinkle 1 teaspoon flour over oil and add fish. Cook about 2 minutes, then turn.

Cut margarine into 6 tiny pieces and add at intervals around sides of pan. Blend lemon juice and wine. Pour around sides of pan and dribble over fish. Simmer gently, uncovered, until liquid is slightly thickened and reduced. Total cooking time should be no more than 5 or 6 minutes.

Transfer fish to warm plates. Add 2 teaspoons of the parsley to pan; stir, and spoon sauce over fish. Sprinkle 2 lemon slices with paprika, the other 2 with the remaining parsley, and decorate fish.

ASPARAGUS MIMOSA

(Each serving, 80 calories)

24 asparagus stalks (depending on size), trimmed and washed

2 teaspoons 100% corn-oil margarine

1 teaspoon lemon juice

½ hard-cooked egg, finely chopped

Steam asparagus over salted water until thick ends are barely tender but color is still brilliant green. Drain and arrange on platter. Dot with margarine, sprinkle with lemon juice, and arrange chopped egg down the center.

STRAWBERRIES MYSTERY

(Each serving, 95 calories)

16 large fresh strawberries

lime or lemon (for grated peel)

2 sprigs fresh mint (optional)

Mystery Sauce Ingredients

¼ teaspoon almond extract

1 teaspoon honey

¼ cup low-fat yogurt

dash of cinnamon

1 teaspoon coffee powder (Turkish, espresso, instant, or ground coffee shaken through fine strainer)

1 kiwi fruit, peeled, or 3 additional large strawberries

Cut stems off berries so they will sit flat, points up, in two shallow dishes.

Put sauce ingredients into blender in order listed and purée. Pour sauce over berries and garnish with additional fruit. Chill. Grate peel liberally over all; add mint.

QUICKIE

VIRGIN MARY COCKTAIL

(Each serving, 25 calories)

A Bloody Mary cocktail without vodka is called a Virgin Mary.

1 cup tomato juice	taste
½ teaspoon lemon juice	2 drops hot-pepper sauce, or more to taste
¼ teaspoon Worcestershire sauce, or more to	2 lemon slices
	4 celery sticks

Blend juices and sauces. Fill glasses with ice; add lemon slices, and insert celery sticks. Pour in juice.

CELERY ROOT AND APPLE SALAD

(Each serving, 100 calories)

Served on crisp butter lettuce, this makes an excellent winter salad. In the summer, substitute hearts of celery.

3 celery roots	mustard
juice of 1 lemon plus 1 tablespoon lemon juice	¼ teaspoon freshly ground white pepper
1 tablespoon mayonnaise (see page 380)	1 Golden Delicious apple
1 teaspoon Dijon	2 tablespoons finely chopped parsley

Wash and peel the celery roots and then grate or chop finely. Sprinkle immediately with lemon juice to prevent discoloration. In a bowl combine the mayonnaise, mustard, 1 tablespoon lemon juice, and pepper and stir with a wire whisk to blend thoroughly. Add dressing to the grated celery. Grate apple and add to salad. Mix together and serve on a bed of lettuce. Sprinkle generously with chopped parsley.

FAST FONDUE
WITH SKINNY DIPPERS

(Each serving, 280 calories for fondue,
150 calories for dippers)

½ clove garlic, cut in pieces
½ cup cold water
2 tablespoons cornstarch
½ cup dry white wine or dry vermouth
¼ pound Swiss, Gruyère, or Monterey Jack cheese, shredded

⅛ teaspoon salt
pepper (preferably white)
½ teaspoon dry mustard

For Dipping:
raw cauliflowerettes
raw mushrooms
raw zucchini sticks
raw broccoli flowerettes
4 Italian bread sticks

Rub a fondue pot or heavy saucepan with garlic. Mix 1 tablespoon or more of the water with cornstarch to make a smooth paste; set aside. Combine wine and remaining water in fondue pot and cook over moderately high heat until liquid is almost boiling. Gradually add cheese, stirring constantly until cheese melts; *do not boil.* Add cornstarch mixture. Continue cooking until fondue begins to thicken. Season with salt, pepper, and mustard. If mixture is not cooked in a fondue pot, transfer to a container that can be placed over a candlewarmer or other heating device at the table. Dip vegetables and bread sticks in fondue to eat.
California Fondue Variation: Use Monterey Jack cheese. Season with crushed dried red chiles or chopped green chiles, either the mild type or fiery *jalapeños.*

PRUNE COMPOTE IN PORT

(Each serving, 185 calories)

In the summer, make this dish with fresh plums.

10 medium-sized prunes	2 thin slices lemon
½ cup port (any type)	1 cinnamon stick, broken in half
¼ cup water	6 whole cloves

Combine all the ingredients in a saucepan, cover, and simmer for about 15 minutes, or until prunes are tender. Serve cold, cool, or warm (with liquid). Divide lemon slices and spices between the two bowls.

Fresh Plum Variation: Use 6 firm purple or red plums. Cut a slit in each so the skin will split attractively. Simmer in the poaching mixture for about 5 minutes, just until plums begin to soften. (Plums contain 5 additional calories per serving.)

BRUNCH OR LATE, LATE SUPPER

RADISHES ON ICE

(Each serving, 55 calories)

12 red radishes with leaves	1 ounce caviar (sturgeon or lumpfish)
1 tray ice, cracked or crushed	

Trim off all but the small inside radish leaves and cut off roots. Fill wide bowl or platter with ice. "Replant" radishes in ice. Fill small dish with caviar and center in the ice. Dip radishes into caviar.

CHIC CONSOMMÉ

(Each serving, 45 calories)

2 cups homemade consommé or chicken broth (see recipe page 383)	2 small bay leaves or 6 very thin slices raw ginger
2 teaspoons sherry	4 whole black peppercorns

Combine all the ingredients and heat through. Serve in wide soup bowls with garnishing spices divided equally.

Note: Add spices just before heating and serving so that flavor does not get too strong.

SVELTE CHICKEN

(Each serving, 205 calories)

1 tablespoon corn oil or olive oil	summer savory (optional) or 1 teaspoon dried rosemary leaves (or 4 long sprigs fresh rosemary)
1 chicken breast, halved and skinless	
salt, pepper, and paprika	
½ teaspoon each oregano and	2 thin slices lemon
	2 small bay leaves

Spread half the oil on the bottom of a small baking pan. Place chicken in pan and brush remaining oil on top.

Sprinkle with salt, pepper, and paprika to color delicately; then add oregano and savory. Lay a lemon slice on each breast and tuck a bay leaf at the side. (Or lay fresh rosemary on, then lemon, and omit bay leaves.)

Bake, uncovered, at 350° F. for about 40 minutes, or until delicate brown but still moist-looking. Serve hot or at room temperature with lemon and herbs still in place.

PEAS AU NATUREL

(Each serving, 65 calories)

½ pound Chinese pea pods or very young peas in pods	⅛ teaspoon salt
	½ teaspoon 100% corn-oil margarine
¾ cup water	

In a small saucepan, combine the whole unshelled pea pods, water, and salt. Cover and simmer about 10 to 15 minutes for green peas; 2 minutes for pea pods. Test a pod with large peas to see if they are soft.

Meanwhile, divide the margarine into 2 small cups on two plates. Drain peas and pile on plates. Pour liquid into cups. Eat pod and all.

CELESTIAL STRAWBERRY ANGEL CAKE

(Each serving, 175 calories)

2 slices angel food cake, each slice 1/12 of an 8-inch cake

¾ cup thinly sliced or crushed strawberries

⅓ cup low-fat yogurt

2 teaspoons brown sugar or kirsch

Garnish: 2 whole strawberries and 2 mint sprigs (optional)

Put each slice of cake in a bowl. Add 2 tablespoons sliced berries to yogurt and spoon rest on cake.

Blend sugar into yogurt, stirring until berries color sauce. Pour over cake. Decorate each with whole berry and a mint sprig. Serve immediately or chill.

DINNER FOR SIX

SMOKED SALMON SPEARS

(Each serving, 55 calories)

6 ounces Nova Scotia or Scotch smoked salmon

12 cucumber spears

freshly ground black pepper

lemon wedges

Cut salmon into 12 lengthwise strips. Wrap each around a cucumber spear. Guests can sprinkle on freshly ground black pepper and lemon juice to taste.

BROILED CHICKEN
WITH MUSTARD SAUCE

(Each serving, 270 calories)

6 chicken-breast halves

3 tablespoons 100% corn-oil margarine, melted

1 tablespoon unbleached flour

1 tablespoon dry mustard

1½ teaspoons fresh or

½ teaspoon dried dill, minced

¼ teaspoon white pepper

¼ teaspoon salt

¾ cup low-fat milk

4 egg yolks, beaten

3 tablespoons lemon juice

Preheat broiler. Place skinless breasts on a rack 5 inches from heat. Brush with half the margarine. Broil for 15 minutes. Turn, brush with remaining margarine and broil another 15 minutes, or until done.

While the chicken is broiling, combine flour, mustard, dill, salt, and pepper in top of double boiler. Combine milk and yolks and stir in. Place over boiling water. Cook, stirring constantly, until mixture thickens. Stir in lemon juice. Spoon sauce over the broiled chicken breasts or other broiled foods such as fish.

GLAZED NEW POTATOES

(Each serving, 90 calories)

6 new potatoes about 3 inches long (white or red-skinned type) or about 1½ pounds

tiny new potatoes

1 tablespoon 100% corn-oil margarine

1 teaspoon honey

Cook unpeeled potatoes in salted water until tender; drain and keep hot. In a saucepan melt margarine, add potatoes, and turn to coat. Dribble in honey and turn just until coated and shiny.

MEDITERRANEAN TOMATO SALAD

(Each serving, 65 calories)

6 large romaine leaves
3 large fully ripe tomatoes, each cut into 4 slices
salt and pepper
6 parsley sprigs
6 lemon wedges
3 tablespoons minced fresh parsley
3 tablespoons chopped green onion
2 tablespoons olive oil

For each serving: Lay a romaine leaf on plate, top with 2 tomato slices, and season with salt and pepper. Tuck a parsley sprig at side and garnish with 1 lemon wedge.

Mix minced parsley with green onion. Sprinkle on tomatoes, then dribble oil on. Squeeze lemon on for tartness desired.

SIMPLY CHEESECAKE

(Each serving, 175 calories)

1½ teaspoons unflavored gelatin
¾ cup cold water
⅓ cup sugar
grated peel of 2 lemons
5 tablespoons fresh lemon juice
2 cups low-fat cottage cheese
1½ teaspoons each rum flavoring and vanilla extract
¾ cup toasted granola or 18 to 24 whole strawberries

In a small saucepan, soften gelatin in water. Heat (but do not simmer), stirring until no gelatin granules are seen on spoon. Cool slightly; pour into blender with lemon peel and juice, cottage cheese, and flavorings. Whirl until lightly whipped. Pour into sherbet glasses. Or, if you want to unmold, use oiled tart pans or ½-cup molds. Chill until firm.

Whirl cereal in blender. At serving time, sprinkle crumbs on top of cheesecake or put 3 or 4 whole strawberries beside each serving.

DRESSINGS AND SAUCES

I present with pride the Golden Door's great, gourmet, low-calorie dressings and sauces. The key to the Golden Door's weight reduction with glorious eating is our collection of very special dressings and sauces which have been developed over the years. We use them to make fresh, simple, and quickly prepared basic foodstuffs even more tasty and elegant.

Use them when lunching and whenever you need dressings or sauces. You will find that we use them throughout the four weeks of dinner menus. The dressings and sauces are listed here alphabetically, according to the principal ingredient or generic term.

BUTTERMILK DRESSING

(Each tablespoon, 15 calories)

3 tablespoons polyunsaturated oil	¼ teaspoon dry English mustard
½ cup low-fat buttermilk	¼ teaspoon salt
3 tablespoons vinegar	⅓ cup peeled, seeded, and diced cucumber
¼ cup catsup (see page 377)	

Place all the ingredients in a bowl and whisk until well blended. Makes 1 cup.

CATSUP

(Each tablespoon, 6 calories)

1 can whole tomatoes (28 ounces)	1 stalk celery, cut into chunks
1 small onion, cut into chunks	6 large parsley sprigs, cut into pieces
1 carrot, cut into chunks	2 teaspoons prepared white horseradish

Purée tomatoes in blender with juice, onion, carrot, celery, and parsley. Blend until smooth. Pour into a saucepan and boil rapidly, uncovered, for 15 minutes, stirring often, or until almost the desired consistency.

Add horseradish and simmer, stirring constantly, until very thick, about 5 minutes longer. Makes 2½ cups.

TIPS: For a very smooth texture, you may blend fully cooked mixture again. Press through a coarse wire strainer to remove seeds and pulp.

For a more traditional catsup, season with 2 teaspoons vinegar and a bit of brown sugar or honey. Fresh tomatoes (2½ pounds) may be substituted if you want less salt. Peel tomatoes before blending by immersing in boiling water for 3 minutes, or until skin strips off easily.

Keep refrigerated. Use within 3 or 4 days. Or freeze small portions to use as needed.

CREAM SAUCE

(Each ½ cup, 80 calories)

2 cups instant nonfat milk	2½ tablespoons unbleached flour
1 tablespoon 100% corn-oil margarine	⅛ teaspoon salt

Bring milk to simmer in a saucepan. In another pan, melt the margarine and blend in the flour and salt, stirring constantly. Remove the flour-margarine mixture from the heat and slowly add the milk, stirring constantly with a wire whisk. Return the sauce to low heat and cook very slowly until mixture thickens. This makes about 2 cups thin cream sauce.

DILL DRESSING

(Each tablespoon, 12 calories)

1 teaspoon Dijon mustard	2 tablespoons water
1 teaspoon Golden Door seasoning salt (see page 381)	2 teaspoons chopped onion
1 teaspoon dried dill	2 teaspoons polyunsaturated oil
1 clove garlic, minced	5 teaspoons wine vinegar

Put mustard and all dry ingredients in a wooden salad bowl. Using a fork, crush everything together well. Add liquids and stir vigorously until well blended.

Serve on any greens with a slightly bitter taste: dandelion greens, endive, chicory, and the like. Makes ½ cup.

HOLLANDAISE

(Each ⅓ cup, 80 calories)

This is a rich, tangy mock hollandaise made without butter.

1 egg yolk	dash of white pepper
¼ cup nonfat milk	1 teaspoon lemon
dash of nutmeg	juice
dash of Golden Door	½ cup plain low-fat
seasoning salt (see	yogurt
page 381)	

In the top of a double boiler, beat the egg yolk with a wire whisk until it turns light yellow. Still beating constantly, very slowly add the nonfat milk which has been blended with nutmeg, seasoning salt, and pepper. Place over boiling water and whisk for a minute before adding lemon juice.

When sauce has thickened, fold in yogurt and heat slightly. Makes ⅔ cup sauce.

LEMON DRESSING

(Each tablespoon, 30 calories)

½ cup polyunsaturated oil	Door seasoning salt (see page 381)
¾ cup water	½ cup low-fat yogurt
¾ cup fresh lemon juice	1 shallot, minced
1 teaspoon Golden	1 clove garlic, minced

Place all ingredients in a blender and blend until smooth. Chill before using. Makes 2½ cups.

MAYONNAISE

(250 calories per recipe; 21 per tablespoon)

1 teaspoon fresh lemon juice
1 raw egg yolk
1 teaspoon Dijon mustard
2 small shallots, or 2 thin onion slices, or a mixture of the two, diced
pinch of salt and white pepper
2 hard-cooked egg yolks
½ cup low-fat yogurt

In a blender, combine the lemon juice, raw egg yolk, mustard, shallots, salt, and pepper. Blend until shallots are puréed. Crumble hard-cooked egg yolks into the container and blend again until creamy. If mix won't purée completely, add 1 or 2 tablespoons of yogurt. Fold egg mixture into yogurt (do not blend—mayonnaise will become too thin). Refrigerate. Will keep at least a week. Makes ¾ cup.

MUSTARD SAUCE

(Each tablespoon, 25 calories)

Excellent with broiled chicken, lamb, cold fish like salmon or tuna, or hot poached or broiled fish. Leftover sauce can be served with vegetables.

1 tablespoon unbleached flour
1 tablespoon dry mustard
1½ teaspoons fresh dill, minced, or ½ teaspoon dried dill weed
¼ teaspoon salt
¼ teaspoon white pepper
¾ cup skim milk
4 egg yolks, beaten
3 tablespoons lemon juice

In the top of a double boiler, combine flour, mustard, dill, salt, and pepper. Stir in milk and yolks. Place over boiling water and cook, stirring constantly, until mixture thickens. Stir in lemon juice. Serve hot. Makes 1 cup.

ORANGE DRESSING FOR FRUIT SALAD

(Each tablespoon, 20 calories)

2 tablespoons honey
¼ cup fresh orange
  juice
1 egg

½ cup low-fat yogurt
pinch of nutmeg and
  salt

Place all ingredients in a blender and whirl until thoroughly mixed. Makes 1 cup.

GOLDEN DOOR SEASONING SALT

This "salt" seasons food beautifully and contributes its own original flavor to cooking.

3 ounces powdered
  vegetable broth
¼ teaspoon garlic
  powder
⅛ teaspoon powdered
  thyme
¼ teaspoon onion
  powder
¼ teaspoon paprika

½ teaspoon powdered
  kelp
⅛ teaspoon ground
  celery seed
¼ teaspoon white
  pepper
¼ teaspoon dry
  mustard

Mix together and store in a closed container in a dry place.

THOUSAND ISLAND DRESSING

(Each tablespoon, 25 calories)

3 tablespoons tomato
  purée
3 tablespoons wine
  vinegar or fresh
  lemon juice
1 cup plain low-fat
  yogurt
1 teaspoon fresh
  horseradish
dash of hot-pepper

sauce
¾ cup chopped chives
3 whole pimientos,
  chopped
3 tablespoons
  polyunsaturated oil
½ cup water
salt to taste
1 hard-cooked egg,
  chopped

Place all the ingredients except egg in blender, and blend until well mixed. Pour dressing into a bowl and fold in chopped egg. Serve at once. Makes about 2 cups.

TIP: As a dip for raw vegetables, add some to plain yogurt.

TOMATO SAUCE

(Each ¼ cup, 40 calories)

Good over fish or ground-beef patties.

1 tablespoon polyunsaturated oil	¾ teaspoon dried oregano
1 clove garlic, finely chopped	3 leaves fresh basil, finely chopped, or
¼ cup chopped onion	½ teaspoon crushed dried basil
1 shallot, finely chopped	2 bay leaves
2 cups tomato purée	2 teaspoons minced parsley
½ cup water	salt and pepper
2 teaspoons fresh oregano, minced, or	

Heat oil in large skillet and sauté garlic, onion, and shallot over medium heat until golden. Add tomato purée, water, and herbs and cook, uncovered, over low heat for 45 minutes, stirring occasionally to prevent sticking. Season with salt and pepper, if necessary. Makes 2 cups.

VEGETARIAN DRESSING DELIGHT

(Each tablespoon, 3 calories)

1 stalk celery, finely chopped	parsley
1 medium-sized tomato, peeled and quartered	¼ cup chopped onion
	1 cup water
	4 tablespoons vinegar
¼ cup chopped chives	2 teaspoons Golden Door seasoning salt
¼ cup chopped	(see page 381)

Place all ingredients in saucepan and bring to boil. Simmer for 5 minutes. Purée in blender. Chill before using. Makes 2 cups.

OUR BASIC BROTH

The classic chicken broth is a real help to fine cooking. Although canned or powdered bouillon may be used in a pinch, the home-prepared broth is infinitely better. Make it ahead when you have time and freeze it in small containers, ready for future use. A vegetarian should prepare a stock broth in a similar manner, but without meat.

CHICKEN BROTH

1 (3-pound) roasting chicken	5 cloves
5 carrots, peeled and cut in chunks	5 peppercorns
	1 teaspoon thyme
5 stalks celery	3 cloves garlic
3 onions	parsley to taste

Place all the ingredients in a large pot with water to cover. Bring to a boil and then reduce heat to a slow simmer. Cook gently for 3 hours. Remove chicken from the pot, strip away the skin, and refrigerate chicken for use in other dishes. Boil broth rapidly for 30 minutes to reduce it. Strain through a sieve lined with cheesecloth. Chill broth and remove congealed fat from the surface before placing broth in storage containers. Freeze, if desired.

BREADS AND SPROUTS

OUR WONDERFUL
WHOLE-WHEAT TECATE BREAD

(Makes 2 loaves—22 slices per loaf,
105 calories per slice)

2 packages yeast	½ cup polyunsaturated
4 cups warm water	oil
(105°-115° F. for dry	7½-8 cups
yeast)	stone-ground
2 tablespoons honey	whole-wheat flour

Place yeast in a very large bowl. Add warm water and stir. Blend in honey and oil. While beating with an electric mixer, add flour gradually until dough pulls off the beaters cleanly. Turn dough out onto a floured board and knead until dough is no longer sticky. To knead, fold the dough toward you and push the outer edge of the dough down, toward you, and then away from you with the heel of your hand. The dough is ready when it is silky and feels slightly bouncy. The kneading will take about 8 to 10 minutes.

Place the dough in an oiled bowl, turning the dough once to oil the top. Cover with a clean cloth and allow to rise in a warm, draft-free spot until doubled in bulk, about 1 hour. (You can check to see if dough is ready by pressing the top with your finger. If a dent remains, the dough has risen enough.)

Punch the dough down; divide it in half and roll each half into a 12- × 15-inch oblong. Starting at the narrow end, roll up, jelly-roll fashion. Seal seam and fold over each end 1 inch. Place, seam side down, in a greased 9- × 5- × 3-inch bread pan. Cover and allow to rise again until doubled in bulk, about 1 hour.

Bake in a preheated 375° F. oven for 50 to 60 minutes, or until the loaf is well browned and has a hollow sound when rapped on top.

Cool bread on racks. To freeze, wrap in moisture- and vapor-proof wrapping paper, pressing out as much air as possible. May be stored, frozen, for about 4 months.

SPROUTS

Use sprouts in both fruit and vegetable salads, in sandwiches, as a garnish, and in homemade bread.

Wheat and many grains and seeds are at their best when sprouted. Nature's own growth processes modify the composition, which results in increased micronutrients, vitamins, and a more digestible protein. Wheat, alfalfa, and mung beans are most widely used for sprouting. However, it is fun to experiment, and soon you can have a year-round table garden in your kitchen.

Soak about a quarter of a cup of seeds overnight. In the morning, rinse in fresh water, drain, and place in an open-mouthed jar covered with cheesecloth or a bit of nylon net. Secure with a rubber band. Lay the jar at a 45° angle so that any surplus moisture will continue to drain. Rinse and drain every morning and evening with slightly warm water to keep the sprouts sweet. In three or four days reap the fruits of your labor. Sprouts can be kept for a day or two in the refrigerator.

SPROUTED BREAKFAST BUNS

I begin every day with one of these buns. To me, they are the staff of life.

2 cups whole-wheat grains, sprout quality	raisins
¾ cup large black	1 heaping tablespoon caraway seeds

Sprout as above 2 cups whole-wheat grains.

Using the finest blade on your electric or hand meat grinder, run the sprouts through twice (once if you have a Champion or similar multi-purpose juicer). Sprinkle over the ground sprouts the raisins and caraway seeds. Mix and form into small buns 3″ in diameter and not over 1½″ thick, or make a flat loaf of the thickness.

Bake on a lightly oiled baking sheet at 350° F. for 50 minutes. Cool and store in refrigerator. Delicious served as is or toasted. Bake fresh buns every few days; because no yeast is used, the buns become very hard in a day or so.

INDEX

ABOUT THE AUTHOR

In 1940, with Edmond Bordeaux Szekely, her former husband, DEBORAH SZEKELY MAZZANTI founded Rancho La Puerta, the first American fitness resort, in Tecate, Baja California. In 1958 she created The Golden Door, hailed as the foremost spa in this country. Born May 3, 1922, in Brooklyn, New York, Deborah Mazzanti was educated in Tahiti, Mexico, and the United States. She is the mother of two children and, with her husband, Dr. Vincent E. Mazzanti, lives in San Diego, California, where she is a highly respected civic leader. Her work on nutrition and fitness has brought her many honors, including appointment in 1975 to President Ford's fifteen-member Committee on Physical Fitness and Sports. She serves on the Board of Trustees of the Menninger Foundation, in Topeka, Kansas, and is Chairman of the Board of Overseers of the University of California at San Diego. In 1977 she was named one of two United States delegates to the International Council on Fitness held at the UNESCO Palace in Paris.